GUIDELINES FOR THE SAFE USE OF WASTEWATER, EXCRETA AND GREYWATER

Volume 4
Excreta and greywater use in agriculture

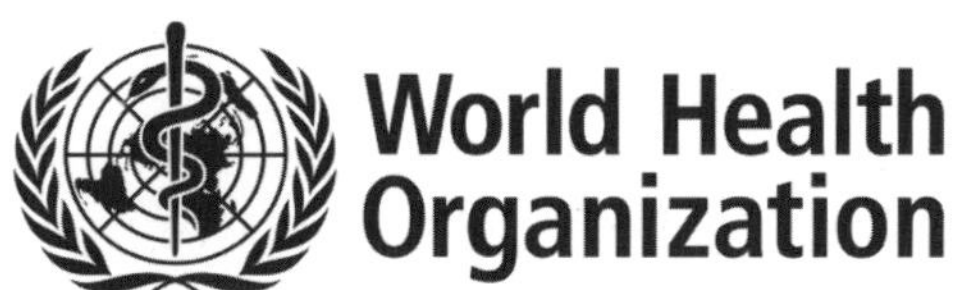

WHO Library Cataloguing-in-Publication Data

WHO guidelines for the safe use of wastewater, excreta and greywater / World Health Organization.

v. 1. Policy and regulatory aspects — v. 2. Wastewater use in agriculture — v. 3. Wastewater and excreta use in aquaculture — v. 4. Excreta and greywater use in agriculture.

1. Water supply. 2. Water supply - legislation. 3. Agriculture. 4. Aquaculture. 5. Sewage. 6. Wastewater treatment plants. 7. Guidelines. I. World Health Organization. II. Title: Safe use of wastewater, excreta and greywater. III. Title: Policy and regulatory aspects. IV. Title: Wastewater use in agriculture. V. Title: Wastewater and excreta use in aquaculture. VI. Title: Excreta and greywater use in agriculture.

ISBN 92 4 154686 7 (set) (NLM classification: WA 675)
ISBN 92 4 154682 4 (v. 1)
ISBN 92 4 154683 2 (v. 2)
ISBN 92 4 154684 0 (v. 3)
ISBN 92 4 154685 9 (v. 4)

Printed in France.

CONTENTS

LIST OF ACRONYMS AND ABBREVIATIONS

AIDS	acquired immunodeficiency syndrome
BKV	BK (polyoma)virus
BOD	biological oxygen demand
BOD_x	x-day biological oxygen demand
cfu	colony forming unit
COD	chemical oxygen demand
DALY	disability adjusted life year
EHEC	enterohaemorrhagic *E. coli*
EIEC	enteroinvasive *E. coli*
EPEC	enteropathogenic *E. coli*
ETEC	enterotoxigenic *E. coli*
FAO	Food and Agriculture Organization of the United Nations
FS	faecal sludge
HIV	human immunodeficiency virus
ID_{50}	median infectious dose
ISO	International Organization for Standardization
JCV	JC (polyoma)virus
MDG	Millennium Development Goal
PHAST	Participatory Hygiene and Sanitation Transformation
P_{inf}	probability of infection
QMRA	quantitative microbial risk assessment
SARAR	Self-esteem, Associative strengths, Resourcefulness, Action-planning, and Responsibility
T_{90}	number of days required for a decimal (90%) reduction (one log reduction)
VIP	ventilated improved pit latrine
VU	viral unit
WHO	World Health Organization
WSSCC	Water Supply and Sanitation Collaborative Council
WTO	World Trade Organization

PREFACE

The United Nations General Assembly (2000) adopted the Millennium Development Goals (MDGs) on 8 September 2000. The MDGs that are most directly related to the safe use of excreta and greywater in agriculture are "Goal 1: Eliminate extreme poverty and hunger" and "Goal 7: Ensure environmental sustainability." The use of excreta and greywater in agriculture can help communities to grow more food and make use of precious water and nutrient resources. However, it should be done safely to maximize public health gains and environmental benefits.

To protect public health and facilitate the rational use of wastewater and excreta in agriculture and aquaculture, in 1973, the World Health Organization (WHO) developed guidelines for wastewater use in agriculture and aquaculture under the title *Reuse of effluents: Methods of wastewater treatment and health safeguards* (WHO, 1973). After a thorough review of epidemiological studies and other information, the guidelines were updated in 1989 as *Health guidelines for the use of wastewater in agriculture and aquaculture* (WHO, 1989). These guidelines have been very influential, and many countries have adopted or adapted them for their wastewater and excreta use practices.

The use of excreta and greywater in agriculture is increasingly considered a method combining water and nutrient recycling, increased household food security and improved nutrition for poor households. Recent interest in excreta and greywater use in agriculture has been driven by water scarcity, lack of availability of nutrients and concerns about health and environmental effects. It was necessary to update the guidelines to take into account scientific evidence concerning pathogens, chemicals and other factors, including changes in population characteristics, changes in sanitation practices, better methods for evaluating risk, social/equity issues and sociocultural practices. There was a particular need to conduct a review of both risk assessment and epidemiological data.

In order to better package the guidelines for appropriate audiences, the third edition of the *Guidelines for the safe use of wastewater, excreta and greywater* is presented in four separate volumes: *Volume 1: Policy and regulatory aspects*; *Volume 2: Wastewater use in agriculture*; *Volume 3: Wastewater and excreta use in aquaculture*; and *Volume 4: Excreta and greywater use in agriculture.*

WHO water-related guidelines are based on scientific consensus and best available evidence; they are developed through broad participation. The *Guidelines for the safe use of wastewater, excreta and greywater* are designed to protect the health of farmers (and their families), local communities and product consumers. They are meant to be adapted to take into consideration national sociocultural, economic and environmental factors. Where the Guidelines relate to technical issues — for example, excreta and greywater treatment — technologies that are readily available and achievable (from both technical and economic standpoints) are explicitly noted, but others are not excluded. Overly strict standards may not be sustainable and, paradoxically, may lead to reduced health protection, because they may be viewed as unachievable under local circumstances and, thus, ignored. The Guidelines therefore strive to maximize overall public health benefits and the beneficial use of scarce resources.

Following an expert meeting in Stockholm, Sweden, WHO published *Water quality: Guidelines, standards and health — Assessment of risk and risk management for water-related infectious disease* (Fewtrell & Bartram, 2001). This document presents a harmonized framework for the development of guidelines and standards for water-related microbial hazards. This framework involves the assessment of health risks prior to the setting of health targets, defining basic control approaches and evaluating the impact of these combined approaches on public health status. The framework is flexible and allows countries to take into consideration health risks that may result from microbial exposures through drinking-water or contact with recreational or occupational water. It is important that health risks from the use of excreta and greywater in agriculture be put into the context of the overall burden of disease within a given population.

This volume of the *Guidelines for the safe use of wastewater, excreta and greywater* provides information on the assessment and management of risks associated with microbial hazards. It explains requirements to promote the safe use of excreta and greywater in agriculture, including minimum procedures and specific health-based targets, and how those requirements are intended to be used. This volume also describes the approaches used in deriving the guidelines, including health-based targets, and includes a substantive revision of approaches to ensuring microbial safety.

This edition of the Guidelines supersedes previous editions (1973 and 1989). The Guidelines are recognized as representing the position of the United Nations system on issues of wastewater, excreta and greywater use and health by "UN-Water," the coordinating body of the 24 United Nations agencies and programmes concerned with water issues. This edition of the Guidelines further develops concepts, approaches and information in previous editions and includes additional information on:

- the context of the overall waterborne disease burden in a population and how the use of excreta and greywater in agriculture may contribute to that burden;
- the Stockholm Framework for development of water-related guidelines and the setting of health-based targets;
- risk analysis;
- risk management strategies, including quantification of different health protection measures;
- guideline implementation strategies.

The revised Guidelines will be useful to all those concerned with issues relating to the safe use of wastewater, excreta and greywater, public health and water and waste management, including environmental and public health scientists, educators, researchers, engineers, policy-makers and those responsible for developing standards and regulations.

ACKNOWLEDGEMENTS

The World Health Organization (WHO) wishes to express its appreciation to all those whose efforts made possible the production of the *Guidelines for the safe use of wastewater, excreta and greywater, Volume 4: Excreta and greywater use in agriculture*, in particular Dr Jamie Bartram (Coordinator, Water, Sanitation and Health, WHO, Geneva), Mr Richard Carr (Technical Officer, Water, Sanitation and Health, WHO, Geneva) and Dr Thor Axel Stenström (Head of Water and Environmental Microbiology, Swedish Institute for Infectious Disease Control, Stockholm), who coordinated the development of this volume.

An international group of experts provided material and participated in the development and review of Volume 4 of the *Guidelines for the safe use of wastewater, excreta and greywater*. Many individuals contributed to each chapter, directly and through associated activities. The contributions[1] of the following to the development of these Guidelines are appreciated:

Mohammad Abed Aziz Al-Rasheed, Ministry of Health, Amman, Jordan
Saqer Al Salem, WHO Regional Centre for Environmental Health Activities, Amman, Jordan
John Anderson, New South Wales Department of Public Works & Services, Sydney, Australia
Andreas Angelakis, National Foundation for Agricultural Research, Institute of Iraklio, Iraklio, Greece
Takashi Asano, University of California at Davis, Davis, California, USA
Nicholas Ashbolt,* University of New South Wales, Sydney, Australia
Lorimer Mark Austin,* Council for Scientific and Industrial Research, Pretoria, South Africa
Ali Akbar Azimi, University of Tehran, Tehran, Iran
Javed Aziz, University of Engineering & Technology, Lahore, Pakistan
Akiça Bahri, National Research Institute for Agricultural Engineering, Water, and Forestry, Ariana, Tunisia
Mohamed Bazza, Food and Agriculture Organization of the United Nations, Cairo, Egypt
Ursula Blumenthal,* London School of Hygiene and Tropical Medicine, London, United Kingdom
Jean Bontoux, University of Montpellier, Montpellier, France
Laurent Bontoux, European Commission, Brussels, Belgium
Robert Bos, WHO, Geneva, Switzerland
Patrik Bracken,* Deutsche Gesellschaft für Technische Zusammenarbeit (GTZ), Eschborn, Germany
François Brissaud, University of Montpellier II, Montpellier, France
Stephanie Buechler, International Water Management Institute, Pantancheru, Andhra Pradesh, India
Paulina Cervantes-Olivier, French Environmental Health Agency, Maisons Alfort, France
Andrew Chang, University of California at Riverside, Riverside, California, USA
Guéladio Cissé, Swiss Centre for Scientific Research, Abidjan, Côte d'Ivoire
Joseph Cotruvo, J. Cotruvo & Associates, Washington, DC, USA
Brian Crathorne, RWE Thames Water, Reading, United Kingdom
David Cunliffe, Environmental Health Service, Adelaide, Australia
Anders Dalsgaard, Royal Veterinary and Agricultural University, Frederiksberg, Denmark

[1] An asterisk (*) indicates the preparation of substantial text inputs.

Gayathri Devi, International Water Management Institute, Andhra Pradesh, India
Jan Olof Drangert,* University of Linköping, Sweden
Pay Drechsel, International Water Management Institute, Accra, Ghana
Bruce Durham, Veolia Water Systems, Derbyshire, United Kingdom
Peter Edwards, Asian Institute of Technology, Klong Luang, Thailand
Dirk Engels, WHO, Geneva, Switzerland
Badri Fattal, The Hebrew University Jerusalem, Jerusalem, Israel
John Fawell, independent consultant, Flackwell Heath, United Kingdom
Pinchas Fine, Institute of Soil, Water and Environmental Sciences, Bet-Dagan, Israel
Jay Fleisher, Nova Southeastern University, Fort Lauderdale, Florida, USA
Yanfen Fu, National Centre for Rural Water Supply Technical Guidance, Beijing, People's Republic of China
Yaya Ganou, Ministry of Health, Ouagadougou, Burkina Faso
Alan Godfrey, United Utilities Water, Warrington, United Kingdom
Maria Isabel Gonzalez Gonzalez, National Institute of Hygiene, Epidemiology and Microbiology, Havana, Cuba
Cagatay Guler, Hacettepe University, Ankara, Turkey
Gary Hartz, Director, Indian Health Service, Rockville, Maryland, USA
Paul Heaton, Power and Water Corporation, Darwin, Northern Territory, Australia
Ivanildo Hespanhol, University of Sao Paolo, Sao Paolo, Brazil
José Hueb, WHO, Geneva, Switzerland
Petter Jenssen,* University of Life Sciences, Aas, Norway
Blanca Jiménez, National Autonomous University of Mexico, Mexico City, Mexico
Jean-François Junger, European Commission, Brussels, Belgium
Ioannis K. Kalavrouziotis, University of Ioannina, Agrinio, Greece
Peter Kolsky, World Bank, Washington, DC, USA
Doulaye Koné,* Swiss Federal Institute for Environmental Science and Technology (EAWAG) / Department of Water and Sanitation in Developing Countries (SANDEC), Duebendorf, Switzerland
Sasha Koo-Oshima, Food and Agriculture Organization of the United Nations, Rome, Italy
Elisabeth Kvarnström,* Verna Ecology Inc., Stockholm, Sweden
Alice Sipiyian Lakati, Department of Environmental Health, Nairobi, Kenya
Valentina Lazarova, ONDEO Services, Le Pecq, France
Pascal Magoarou, European Commission, Brussels, Belgium
Duncan Mara,* University of Leeds, Leeds, United Kingdom
Gerardo Mogol, Department of Health, Manila, Philippines
Gerald Moy, WHO, Geneva, Switzerland
Rafael Mujeriego, Technical University of Catalonia, Barcelona, Spain
Constantino Nurizzo, Politecnico di Milano, Milan, Italy
Gideon Oron, Ben-Gurion University of the Negev, Kiryat Sde-Boker, Israel
Mohamed Ouahdi, Ministry of Health and Population, Algiers, Algeria
Albert Page, University of California at Riverside, Riverside, California, USA
Genxing Pan, Nanjing Agricultural University, Nanjing, People's Republic of China
Nikolaos Paranychianakis, National Foundation for Agricultural Research, Institute of Iraklio, Iraklio, Greece
Martin Parkes, North China College of Water Conservancy and Hydropower, Zhengzhou, Henan, People's Republic of China

Anne Peasey, Imperial College (formerly with London School of Hygiene and Tropical Medicine), London, United Kingdom
Susan Petterson,* University of New South Wales, Sydney, Australia
Liqa Raschid-Sally, International Water Management Institute, Accra, Ghana
Anna Richert-Stinzing,* Verna Ecology Inc,, Stockholm, Sweden
Kerstin Röske, Institute for Medicine, Microbiology and Hygiene, Dresden, Germany
Lorenzo Savioli, WHO, Geneva, Switzerland
Jørgen Schlundt, WHO, Geneva, Switzerland
Caroline Schönning,* Swedish Institute for Infectious Disease Control, Stockholm, Sweden
Janine Schwartzbrod, University of Nancy, Nancy, France
Louis Schwartzbrod, University of Nancy, Nancy, France
Natalia Shapirova, Ministry of Health, Tashkent, Uzbekistan
Hillel Shuval, The Hebrew University of Jerusalem, Jerusalem, Israel
Martin Strauss,* Swiss Federal Institute for Environmental Science and Technology (EAWAG) / Department of Water and Sanitation in Developing Countries (SANDEC), Duebendorf, Switzerland
Ted Thairs, EUREAU Working Group on Wastewater Reuse (former Secretary), Herefordshire, United Kingdom
Terrence Thompson, WHO Regional Office for the Western Pacific, Manila, Philippines
Sarah Tibatemwa, National Water & Sewerage Corporation, Kampala, Uganda
Andrea Tilche, European Commission, Brussels, Belgium
Mwakio P. Tole, Kenyatta University, Nairobi, Kenya
Francisco Torrella, University of Murcia, Murcia, Spain
Hajime Toyofuku, WHO, Geneva, Switzerland
Wim van der Hoek, independent consultant, Landsmeer, The Netherlands
Johan Verink, ICY Waste Water & Energy, Hanover, Germany
Marcos von Sperling, Federal University of Minas Gerais, Belo Horizonte, Brazil
Christine Werner,* Deutsche Gesellschaft für Technische Zusammenarbeit (GTZ), Eschborn, Germany
Steve White, RWE Thames Water, Reading, United Kingdom

Thanks are also due to Marla Sheffer for editing the complete text of the Guidelines, Windy Prohom and Colette Desigaud for their assistance in project administration and Peter Gosling, who acted as the rapporteur for the Final Review Meeting for the Finalization of the Third Edition of the WHO Guidelines for the Safe Use of Wastewater, Excreta and Greywater in Geneva.

The preparation of these Guidelines would not have been possible without the generous support of the United Kingdom Department for International Development, the Swedish International Development Cooperation Agency (Sida) through the Stockholm Environment Institute, the Norwegian Ministry of Foreign Affairs, the Deutsche Gesellschaft für Technische Zusammenarbeit (GTZ) and the Dutch Ministry of Foreign Affairs (DGIS) through WASTE (advisors on urban environment and development).

EXECUTIVE SUMMARY

This volume of the World Health Organization's (WHO) *Guidelines for the safe use of wastewater, excreta and greywater* describes the present state of knowledge regarding the impact of excreta and greywater use in agriculture on the health of product consumers, workers and their families and local communities. Health hazards are identified for each group at risk, and appropriate health protection measures to mitigate the risks are discussed.

The primary aim of the Guidelines is to maximize public health protection and the beneficial use of important resources. The purpose of this volume is to ensure that the use of excreta and greywater in agriculture is made as safe as possible so that the nutritional and household food security benefits can be shared widely in affected communities. Thus, the adverse health impacts of excreta and greywater use in agriculture should be carefully weighed against the benefits to health and the environment associated with these practices. Yet this is not a matter of simple trade-offs. Wherever excreta and greywater use contributes significantly to food security and nutritional status, the point is to identify associated hazards, define the risks they represent to vulnerable groups and design measures aimed at reducing these risks.

This volume of the Guidelines is intended to be used as the basis for the development of international and national approaches (including standards and regulations) to managing the health risks from hazards associated with excreta and greywater use in agriculture, as well as providing a framework for national and local decision-making.

The information provided is applicable to the intentional use of excreta and greywater in agriculture, but it should also be relevant to their unintentional use.

The Guidelines provide an integrated preventive management framework for safety applied from the point of household excreta and greywater generation to the consumption of products grown with treated excreta applied as fertilizers or treated greywater used for irrigation purposes. They describe reasonable minimum requirements of good practice to protect the health of the people using treated excreta or greywater or consuming products grown with these for fertilization or irrigation purposes and provide information that is then used to derive health-based targets. Neither the minimum good practices nor the health-based targets are mandatory limits. The preferred approaches adopted by national or local authorities towards implementation of the Guidelines, including health-based targets, may vary depending on local social, cultural, environmental and economic conditions, as well as knowledge of routes of exposure, the nature and severity of hazards and the effectiveness of health protection measures available.

The revised *Guidelines for the safe use of wastewater, excreta and greywater* will be useful to all those concerned with issues relating to the safe use of wastewater, excreta and greywater, public health, water resources development and wastewater management. The target audience may include public health, agricultural and environmental scientists, agriculture professionals, educators, researchers, engineers, policy-makers and those responsible for developing standards and regulations.

Introduction

Traditional waterborne sewerage will continue to dominate sanitation for the foreseeable future. Since only a fraction of existing wastewater treatment plants in the world are optimally reducing levels of pathogenic microorganisms and since a majority of people living in both rural and urban areas will not be connected to centralized wastewater treatment systems, alternative sanitation approaches need to be developed in parallel.

The United Nations General Assembly adopted the Millennium Development Goals (MDGs) on 8 September 2000 (United Nations General Assembly, 2000). The MDGs most directly related to the use of excreta and greywater in agriculture are "Goal 1: Eliminate extreme poverty and hunger" and "Goal 7: Ensure environmental sustainability." The sanitation target in Goal 7 is to halve, by 2015, the proportion of people without access to adequate sanitation. Household- or community-centred source separation is one of the alternative approaches that is rapidly expanding in order to meet this target. It also helps to prevent environmental degradation and to promote sustainable recycling of the existing plant nutrients in human excreta for food production.

The principal forces driving the increase in use of excreta and greywater in agriculture are:

- increasing water scarcity and stress, and degradation of freshwater resources resulting from the improper disposal of wastewater, excreta and greywater;
- population increase and related increased demand for food and fibre;
- a growing recognition of the resource value of excreta and the nutrients it contains;
- the MDGs, especially the goals for ensuring environmental sustainability and eliminating poverty and hunger.

Growing competition between agricultural and urban areas for high-quality freshwater supplies, particularly in arid, semi-arid and densely populated regions, will increase the pressure on this increasingly scarce resource. Most population growth is expected to occur in urban and periurban areas in developing countries (United Nations Population Division, 2002). Population growth increases both the demand for fresh water and the amount of wastes that are discharged into the environment, thus leading to more pollution of clean water sources. Household-centred source separation and the safe use of excreta and greywater in agriculture will help to alleviate these pressures and help communities to grow more food and conserve precious water and nutrient resources. The additional advantages of nutrient use from excreta as fertilizers are that this "product" is less contaminated with industrial chemicals than when wastewater is used and that it saves water for other uses.

This volume focuses mainly on small-scale applications. It is applicable to both industrialized and developing countries.

The Stockholm Framework

The Stockholm Framework is an integrated approach that combines risk assessment and risk management to control water-related diseases. This provides a harmonized framework for the development of health-based guidelines and standards in terms of water- and sanitation-related microbial hazards. The Stockholm Framework involves the assessment of health risks prior to the setting of health-based targets and the development of guideline values, defining basic control approaches and evaluating the impact of these combined approaches on public health. The Stockholm Framework provides the conceptual framework for these Guidelines and other WHO water-related guidelines.

Assessment of health risk

Three types of evaluations are used to assess risk: microbial analysis, epidemiological studies and quantitative microbial risk assessment (QMRA). Human faeces contain a variety of different pathogens, reflecting the prevalence of infection in the population; in contrast, only a few pathogenic species may be excreted in urine. The risks associated with both reuse of urine as a fertilizer and the use of greywater for irrigation purposes are related to cross-contamination by faecal matter. Epidemiological data for the assessment of risk through treated faeces, faecal sludge, urine or greywater are scarce and unreliable, while ample evidence exists related to untreated faecal matter. In addition, microbial analyses are partly unreliable in the prediction of risk due to a more rapid die-off of indicator organisms such as *Escherichia coli* in urine, leading to an underestimation of the risk of pathogen transmission. The opposite may occur in greywater, where a growth of the indicator bacteria on easily degradable organic substances may lead to an overestimation of the risks. Based on the above limitations, QMRA is the main approach taken, due to the range of organisms with common transmission characteristics and their prevalence in the population. Factors accounted for include:

- epidemiological features (including infectious dose, latency, hosts and intermediate host);
- persistence in different environments outside the human body (and potential for growth);
- major transmission routes;
- relative efficiency of different treatment barriers;
- risk management measures.

Health-based targets

Health-based targets define a level of health protection that is relevant to each hazard. A health-based target can be based on a standard metric of disease, such as a disability adjusted life year or DALY (i.e. 10^{-6} DALY), or it can be based on an appropriate health outcome, such as the prevention of exposure to pathogens in excreta and greywater anytime between their generation at the household level and their use in agriculture. To achieve a health-based target, health protection measures are developed. Usually a health-based target can be achieved by combining health protection measures targeted at different steps in the process.

The health-based targets may be achieved through different treatment barriers or health protection measures. The barriers relate to verification monitoring, mainly in large-scale systems, as illustrated in Table 1 for excreta and greywater. Verification monitoring is not applicable to urine.

The health-based targets may also relate to operational monitoring, such as storage as an on-site treatment measure or further treatment off-site after collection. This is exemplified for faeces from small-scale systems in Table 2.

For collected urine, storage criteria apply that are derived mainly from compiled risk assessment studies. The information obtained has been converted to operational guidelines to limit the risk to a level below 10^{-6} DALY, also accounting for additional health protection measures. The operational guidelines are based on source separation of urine (Table 3). In case of heavy faecal cross-contamination, the suggested storage times may be lengthened. If urine is used as a fertilizer of crops for household consumption only, it can be used directly without storage. The likelihood of household disease transmission attributable to the lack of hygiene is much higher than that of transmission through urine applied as a fertilizer.

Table 1. Guideline values for verification monitoring in large-scale treatment systems of greywater, excreta and faecal sludge for use in agriculture

	Helminth eggs (number per gram total solids or per litre)	*E. co li* (number per 100 ml)
Treated faeces and faecal sludge	<1/g total solids	<1000 g/total solids
Greywater for use in:		
• Restricted irrigation	<1/litre	$<10^5$ [a] Relaxed to $<10^6$ when exposure is limited or regrowth is likely
• Unrestricted irrigation of crops eaten raw	<1/litre	$<10^3$ Relaxed to $<10^4$ for high-growing leaf crops or drip irrigation

[a] These values are acceptable due to the regrowth potential of *E. coli* and other faecal coliforms in greywater.

Table 2. Recommendations for storage treatment of dry excreta and faecal sludge before use at the household and municipal levels[a]

Treatment	Criteria	Comment
Storage; ambient temperature 2–20 °C	1.5–2 years	Will eliminate bacterial pathogens; regrowth of *E. coli* and *Salmonella* may need to be considered if rewetted; will reduce viruses and parasitic protozoa below risk levels. Some soil-borne ova may persist in low numbers.
Storage; ambient temperature >20–35 °C	>1 year	Substantial to total inactivation of viruses, bacteria and protozoa; inactivation of schistosome eggs (<1 month); inactivation of nematode (roundworm) eggs, e.g. hookworm (*Ancylostoma*/*Necator*) and whipworm (*Trichuris*); survival of a certain percentage (10–30%) of *Ascaris* eggs (≥4 months), whereas a more or less complete inactivation of *Ascaris* eggs will occur within 1 year.
Alkaline treatment	pH >9 during >6 months	If temperature >35 °C and moisture <25%, lower pH and/or wetter material will prolong the time for absolute elimination.

[a] No addition of new material.

For all types of treated excreta, additional safety measures apply. These include, for example, a recommended withholding time of one month between the moment of application of the treated excreta as a fertilizer and the time of crop harvest (Figure 1). Based on QMRA, this time period has been shown to result in a probability of infection well below 10^{-4}, which is within the range of a 10^{-6} DALY level.

Health protection measures

A variety of health protection measures can be used to reduce health risks for local communities, workers and their families and for the consumers of the fertilized or irrigated products.

Hazards associated with the consumption of excreta-fertilized products include excreta-related pathogens. The risk from infectious diseases is significantly reduced if foods are eaten after proper handling and adequate cooking. The following health protection measures have an impact on product consumers:

- excreta and greywater treatment;
- crop restriction;
- waste application and withholding periods between fertilization and harvest to allow die-off of remaining pathogens;
- hygienic food handling and food preparation practices;
- health and hygiene promotion;
- produce washing, disinfection and cooking.

Table 3. Recommended storage times for urine mixture[a] based on estimated pathogen content[b] and recommended crops for larger systems[c]

Storage temperature (°C)	Storage time (months)	Possible pathogens in the urine mixture after storage	Recommended crops
4	≥1	Viruses, protozoa	Food and fodder crops that are to be processed
4	≥6	Viruses	Food crops that are to be processed, fodder crops[d]
20	≥1	Viruses	Food crops that are to be processed, fodder crops[d]
20	≥6	Probably none	All crops[e]

[a] Urine or urine and water. When diluted, it is assumed that the urine mixture has a pH of at least 8.8 and a nitrogen concentration of at least 1 g/l.

[b] Gram-positive bacteria and spore-forming bacteria are not included in the underlying risk assessments, but are not normally recognized as a cause of any infections of concern.

[c] A larger system in this case is a system where the urine mixture is used to fertilize crops that will be consumed by individuals other than members of the household from whom the urine was collected.

[d] Not grasslands for production of fodder.

[e] For food crops that are consumed raw, it is recommended that the urine be applied at least one month before harvesting and that it be incorporated into the ground if the edible parts grow above the soil surface.

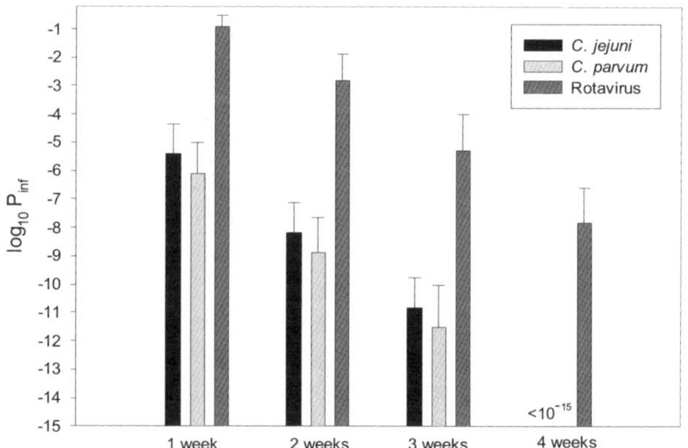

Figure 1

Mean probability of infection by pathogens following ingestion of crops fertilized with unstored urine with varying withholding periods (P_{inf} = probability of infection)

For all types of treated excreta, additional safety measures apply. These include, for example, a recommended withholding time of one month between the moment of application of the treated excreta as a fertilizer and the time of crop harvest (Figure 1). Based on QMRA, this time period has been shown to result in a probability of infection well below 10^{-4}, which is within the range of a 10^{-6} DALY level.

Workers and their families may be exposed to excreta-related and vector-borne pathogens (in certain locations) through excreta and greywater use activities. Excreta and greywater treatment is a measure to prevent diseases associated with excreta and greywater but will not directly impact vector-borne diseases. Other health protection measures for workers and their families include:

- use of personal protective equipment;
- access to safe drinking-water and sanitation facilities at farms;
- health and hygiene promotion;
- disease vector and intermediate host control;
- reduced vector contact.

Local communities are at risk from the same hazards as workers. If they do not have access to safe drinking-water, they may use contaminated irrigation water for drinking or for domestic purposes. Children may also play or swim in the contaminated water. Similarly, if the activities result in increased vector breeding, then vector-borne diseases can affect local communities, even if they do not have direct access to the fields. To reduce health hazards, the following health protection measures for local communities may be used:

- excreta and greywater treatment;
- limited contact during handling and controlled access to fields;
- access to safe drinking-water and sanitation facilities in local communities;
- health and hygiene promotion;
- disease vector and intermediate host control;
- reduced vector contact.

Monitoring and system assessment

Monitoring has three different purposes: validation, or proving that the system is capable of meeting its design requirements; operational monitoring, which provides information regarding the functioning of individual components of the health protection measures; and verification, which usually takes place at the end of the process to ensure that the system is achieving the specified targets.

The three functions of monitoring are each used for different purposes at different times. Validation is performed when a new system is developed or when new processes are added and is used to test or prove that the system is capable of meeting the specified targets. Operational monitoring is used on a routine basis to indicate that processes are working as expected. Monitoring of this type relies on simple measurements that can be read quickly so that decisions can be made in time to remedy a problem. Verification is used to show that the end product (e.g. treated excreta or greywater; crops) meets treatment targets and ultimately the health-based targets. Information from verification monitoring is collected periodically and thus would arrive too late to allow managers to make decisions to prevent a hazard break-through. However, verification monitoring in larger systems can indicate trends over time (e.g. if the efficiency of a specific process was improving or decreasing).

The most effective means of consistently ensuring safety in the agricultural use of excreta and greywater is through the use of a comprehensive risk assessment and risk management approach that encompasses all steps in the process from waste generation to treatment, use of excreta as fertilizers or use of greywater for irrigation purposes and product use or consumption. Three components of this approach are important for achieving the health-based targets: system assessment, identifying control measures and methods for monitoring them and developing a management plan.

Sociocultural aspects

Human behavioural patterns are a key determining factor in the transmission of excreta-related diseases. The social feasibility of changing certain behavioural patterns in order to introduce excreta or greywater use schemes or to reduce disease transmission in existing schemes needs to be assessed on an individual project basis. Cultural beliefs and public perceptions of excreta and greywater use vary so widely in different parts of the world that one cannot assume that any of the local practices that have evolved in relation to such use can be readily transferred elsewhere. Even when projects are technically well planned and all of the relevant health protection measures have been included, they can fail if cultural beliefs and public perceptions have not been adequately accounted for.

Environmental aspects

Excreta are an important source of nutrients for many farmers. The direct use of excreta and greywater on arable land tends to minimize the environmental impact in both the local and global context. Reuse of excreta on arable land secures valuable fertilizers for crop production and limits the negative impact on water bodies. The environmental impact of different sanitation systems can be measured in terms of the conservation and use of natural resources, discharges to water bodies, air emissions and the impacts on soils. In this type of assessment, source separation and household-centred use systems frequently score more favourably than conventional systems.

Application of excreta and greywater to agricultural land will reduce the direct impacts on water bodies. As for any type of fertilizer, however, the nutrients may percolate into the groundwater if applied in excess or flushed into the surface water after excessive rainfall. This impact will always be less than that of the direct use of water bodies as the primary recipient of excreta and greywater. Surface water bodies are affected by agricultural drainage and runoff. Impacts depend on the type of water body (rivers, agricultural channels, lakes or dams) and their use, as well as the hydraulic retention time and the function it performs within the ecosystem.

Phosphorus is an essential element for plant growth, and external phosphorus from mined phosphate is usually supplied in agriculture in order to increase plant productivity. World supplies of accessible mined phosphate are diminishing. Approximately 25% of the mined phosphorus ends up in aquatic environments or is buried in landfills or other sinks. This discharge into aquatic environments is damaging, as it causes eutrophication of water bodies. Urine alone contains more than 50% of the phosphorus excreted by humans. Thus, the diversion and use of urine in agriculture can aid crop production and reduce the costs of and need for advanced wastewater treatment processes to remove phosphorus from the treated effluents.

Economic and financial considerations

Economic factors are especially important when the viability of a new project is appraised, but even an economically worthwhile project can fail without careful financial planning.

Economic analysis and financial considerations are crucial for encouraging the safe use of excreta. Economic analysis seeks to establish the feasibility of a project and enables comparisons between different options. The cost transfers to other sectors (e.g. the health and environmental impacts on downstream communities) also need to be included in a cost analysis. This can be facilitated by the use of multiple-objective decision-making processes.

Financial planning considers how the project is to be paid for. In establishing the financial feasibility of a project, it is important to determine the sources of revenues and clarify who will pay for what. The ability to profitably sell products fertilized with excreta or irrigated with greywater also needs analysis.

Policy aspects

Appropriate policies, legislation, institutional frameworks and regulations at the international, national and local levels facilitate safe excreta and greywater management practices. In many countries where such practices take place, these frameworks and regulations are lacking.

Policy is the set of procedures, rules, decision-making criteria and allocation mechanisms that provide the basis for programmes and services. Policies set priorities, and associated strategies allocate resources for their implementation. Policies are implemented through four types of instruments: laws and regulations; economic measures; information and education programmes; and assignments of rights and responsibilities for providing services.

In developing a national policy framework to facilitate the safe use of excreta as fertilizer, it is important to define the objectives of the policy, assess the current policy environment and develop a national approach. National approaches for adequate sanitation based on the WHO Guidelines will protect public health optimally when they are integrated into comprehensive public health programmes that include other sanitary measures, such as health and hygiene promotion and improving access to safe drinking-water.

National approaches need to be adapted to the local sociocultural, environmental and economic circumstances, but they should be aimed at progressive improvement of public health. Interventions that address the greatest local health threats first should be given the highest priority. As resources and new data become available, additional health protection measures can be introduced.

Planning and implementation periode

Planning and implementation of programmes for the agricultural use of excreta and greywater require a comprehensive, progressive and incremental approach that responds to the greatest health priorities first. This integrated approach should be based on an assessment of the current sanitary situation and should take into account the local aspects related to water supply and solid waste management. A sound basis for such an approach can be found in the Bellagio Principles, which prescribe that stakeholders be provided with the relevant information, enabling them to make "informed choices." Thus, a wider range of decision-making and evaluation criteria for sanitation services can be applied.

In addition, project planning requires consideration of several different issues, identified through the involvement of stakeholders applying participatory methods and considering treatment, crop restriction, waste application, human exposure control, costs, technical aspects, support services and training both for risk reduction and for maximizing the benefits from an individual as well as a community point of view.

1 INTRODUCTION

This volume of the *Guidelines for the safe use of wastewater, excreta and greywater* presents information on the health risks associated with pathogens that occur in human excreta and greywater when used in agriculture. It also presents health protection measures, including technical barriers and best practices to minimize these risks. The Guidelines are based on the development and use of health-based targets. Health-based targets establish a goal of attaining a certain level of health protection in an exposed population. This volume furthermore includes evidence on the fertilizing value of treated excreta, relates their use to sustainability criteria, outlines planning, prevention and implementation strategies and puts their safe handling in a legal, institutional and economic framework. Any possible adverse impacts will be weighed against the health and environmental benefits of recirculating nutrients to arable land. Positive health impacts, such as the contribution to better nutrition and the impact on household food security, especially for the poor, need to be considered in this context.

The poor bear the heaviest burden of diseases transmitted through faecal–oral pathways, which include contaminated water and improper excreta disposal. Therefore, the positive health outcome of these Guidelines is potentially greatest for the poorest members of society, reflecting a social equity dimension. A significant amount of human excreta is used in subsistence agriculture. Although the main focus of the Guidelines is on small-scale systems, their scope is not limited to these.

This volume of the *Guidelines for the safe use of wastewater, excreta and greywater* is structured as outlined in Figure 1.1.

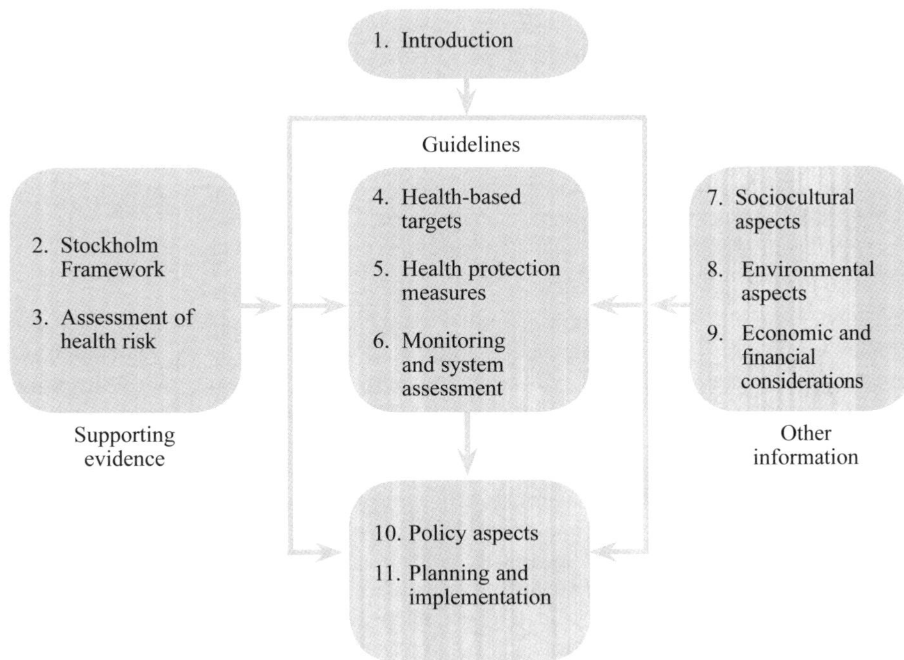

Figure 1.1
Structure of Volume 4 of the *Guidelines for the safe use of wastewater, excreta and greywater*

Chapter 1 presents the objectives and introduces some conceptual issues; it also describes the target audience, the driving forces behind excreta and greywater use, the resource value and the Millennium Development Goals (MDGs). Chapter 2 provides an overview of the Stockholm Framework. Chapter 3 provides the epidemiological, microbiological and risk assessment bases for the Guidelines. Chapters 4 and 5 present health-based targets and health protection measures, including technical components, crop restrictions, agricultural methods, human exposure control, hygiene education and health care aspects, while chapter 6 provide practical guidance on monitoring and system assessment. Chapters 7, 8 and 9 provide background information on sociocultural, environmental and economic and financial aspects. The policy, institutional and legal frameworks are covered in chapter 10, and planning and implementation procedures are presented in chapter 11.

1.1 Objectives and general considerations

The primary objective of these Guidelines is to protect the health of individuals and benefit the health status of communities by the safe use of excreta and greywater in a range of agricultural applications. The Guidelines consider the positive health outcomes of this use (such as its contribution to better nutrition and food security), without presenting these as trade-offs.

To this end, the Guidelines describe recommended reasonable minimum safe practice requirements and system performance to protect the health of the people using excreta and greywater, local communities and the consumers of products grown with them. The Guidelines support the development and implementation of risk management strategies. The required level of health protection can be achieved by using a combination of management approaches (e.g. handling and crop restriction, human exposure control) and quality targets to arrive at the specified health outcome. Thus, the guidance provided concerns both good handling practices and quality speculations and may include:

- a level of management;
- a concentration of a constituent that does not represent a significant risk to the health of members of important user groups;
- a condition under which such exposures are unlikely to occur; or
- a combination of the last two.

The Guidelines relate to an integrated risk management framework (see the Stockholm Framework in chapter 2) applied from the point of generation to consumption of products grown with excreta or greywater. The approach followed in these Guidelines is intended to lead to national standards and regulations that can be readily implemented and enforced and are protective of public health. It is essential that each country review its needs and capacities in developing a regulatory framework. In order to define national standards and procedures, it is necessary to consider the Guidelines in the context of local environmental, social, economic and cultural conditions (WHO, 2004a). Successful implementation of the Guidelines will require a broad-based policy framework that includes positive and negative incentives to alter behaviour and monitor and improve situations. This will require significant efforts in intersectoral coordination and cooperation at national and local levels and the development of suitable skills and expertise.

In some situations, it will not be possible to fully implement the Guidelines at once. The Guidelines allow incremental implementation. The greatest threats to health should be given the highest priority and addressed first. Over time, it should be possible to adjust the risk management framework to strive for the continual improvement of public health.

Ultimately, the judgement of safety — or what is a tolerable level of risk in particular circumstances — is a matter in which society as a whole has a role to play. The final judgement as to whether the benefit from using any of the Guidelines and guideline values as national or local standards justifies the cost is for each country to decide, in the context of national public health, environmental and socioeconomic realities and international trade regulations. The final judgement on safety standards and procedures is a matter for broad public consultation and should result from a transparent and accountable political decision-making process.

1.2 Target audience and definitions

These Guidelines are targeted at decision-makers and regulators in World Health Organization (WHO) Member States who are responsible for setting the framework for, planning and implementing activities in sanitation-related areas. It is hoped that these Guidelines will also be useful to all those with a stake or interest in the safe use of excreta and greywater, public health and water and waste management, including environmental and public health scientists, educators, farmers, researchers, engineers, community planners, policymakers and regulators.

The health hazards linked to the agricultural use of excreta and greywater vary with the distribution of pathogens, the local transmission and exposure pathways and the capacity of health services to deal with them. The pathways are closely related to handling practices in the chain from the producer to the use, including ingestion of contaminated food products. The responsibility for minimizing health risks lies with the direct users of excreta and greywater, with the planners and managers of systems where excreta and greywater are applied and with the local and national regulatory authorities that set standards for norms and procedures. Nongovernmental organizations and special interest groups also have an important role to play in helping local communities to maximize the reuse of valuable resources while ensuring that health risks are reduced to a minimum.

In the context of these Guidelines, "excreta" refers to faeces and urine, but also to excreta-derived products, such as faecal sludge and septage (for definitions of terms used in the Guidelines, see Annex 1). Sludge derived from the treatment of municipal or industrial wastewater is not included in these guidelines. The main focus of these Guidelines is the prevention of infectious disease transmission, and health issues associated with exposure to chemicals are discussed only in broad terms.

"Greywater" is defined as wastewater from the kitchen, bath and laundry, excluding wastewater from toilets, and therefore generally contains lower concentrations of excreta, except in specific situations as a result of infant care or where anal cleansing water is combined with the greywater. Greywater is used mainly for irrigation, but health issues are also associated with the use of greywater for other purposes, such as toilet flushing, service water or groundwater infiltration.

1.3 International guidelines and national standards

1.3.1 National standards

WHO Guidelines are intended to provide a consistent level of health protection in different settings, and they should be adapted for implementation under specific environmental, sociocultural and economic conditions at the national level or below. In some cases, countries may choose to develop different standards for products consumed locally and for products destined for export. Wherever lower national standards are set, based on a locally adopted level of tolerable risk (see chapter 2 for a further discussion of tolerable risk), the incidence of diarrhoeal or other diseases needs to be accounted for.

1.3.2 Food exports

The Guidelines can be adapted based on local conditions, except in relation to the rules that govern international trade in food, which have been agreed during the Uruguay Round of Multilateral Trade Negotiations and apply to all members of the World Trade Organization (WTO). With regard to food safety, rules are set out in the Agreement on the Application of Sanitary and Phytosanitary Measures. According to this, WTO members have the right to take legitimate measures to protect the life and health of their populations from hazards in food, provided that the measures are not unjustifiably restrictive of trade (WHO, 1999). There are documented cases where the import of contaminated vegetables has led to disease outbreaks in recipient countries. Pathogens can be introduced into communities lacking immunity, resulting in important disease outbreaks (Frost et al., 1995; Kapperud et al., 1995). Guidelines for the international trade of excreta-fertilized and wastewater-irrigated food products therefore need to be based on sound scientific risk management principles.

WHO Guidelines for the safe use of excreta and greywater in agriculture are based on a risk analysis approach that is recognized as the fundamental methodology underlying the development of food safety standards that both provide adequate health protection and facilitate trade in food. Adherence to the WHO Guidelines will help to ensure the international trade of safe food products in the case of export of excreta-fertilized or greywater-irrigated food products.

1.4 Factors that affect sustainability in sanitation

Sustainable development, as defined in the Report of the World Commission on Environment and Development (WCED, 1987), is development that "meets the needs of the present generation without compromising the ability of future generations to meet their own needs." From both a sustainability and a public health perspective, increasing access to adequate sanitation and promoting the adoption by individuals and communities of key hygienic behaviours are first priorities.

Within the scope of the *Guidelines for the safe use of wastewater, excreta and greywater*, sustainability can be described as the ability to plan and manage the use of excreta and greywater in agriculture as important resources in such a way that human health is not compromised, nutrients are recycled for food production and negative impacts on water resources or the environment are avoided. Sustainability needs to be defined in relation to the interaction of users, organizational structure and technology, with a range of important criteria: health and hygiene, environmental and resource use, economy, sociocultural aspects and use and technology function. These aspects should be addressed with appropriate policies and within a conducive legal and regulatory framework; they are covered in different parts of the Guidelines.

1.4.1 Health and hygiene

The process of reducing disease burdens through improved sanitation is associated with the determinants of sustainability and is closely related to hygiene, behavioural change and proper access to and use of water and sanitation facilities. Focusing on just the provision of sanitation hardware will not result in sustainable change and will therefore not have a lasting impact on the health status of communities. Health aspects of excreta and greywater use are further dealt with in chapters 3 and 5.

1.4.2 Environment and resource use

Minimizing the negative impacts of excreta and greywater on surface water and groundwater and making more efficient use of the nutrient resources that they contain for crop and energy production will directly contribute to environmental sustainability. The environment will most importantly benefit from the treatment and safe use of excreta and greywater in terms of:

- recycling of water and nutrient resources;
- reduction of pressure on freshwater resources;
- reduction of downstream pollution from the discharge of wastes;
- reduction of potential environmental impacts from various chemicals (among others, endocrine disruptors, pharmaceuticals and their residues, which partly adsorb to soil particles and/or biodegrade in the soil, reducing the environmental impact on waters).

Environmental aspects of excreta and greywater use are further discussed in chapter 8.

1.4.3 Economy

Economic aspects of sanitation are important at both national and household levels. At the national level, planners want to ensure optimal cost-effectiveness of investments in hygiene and sanitation options. These investments should give substantial economic returns in health benefits and time savings (Hutton & Haller, 2004). The cost–benefit of reducing adverse health and other impacts downstream as a result of better wastewater treatment and/or reducing waste discharges into surface waters has not been estimated but is likely to be as important.

Several studies have indicated that it is more cost-effective to provide funding for creating sanitation and hygiene demand through promotion than to heavily subsidize sanitation hardware (Cairncross, 1992; Wright, 1997; Samanta & van Wijk, 1998; Kolsky & Diop 2004). Most costs associated with gaining access to sanitation are incurred at the household level. Consumers want products that are durable and that will not cost a lot to operate and maintain. It is unlikely that sanitation will become sustainable unless local resources are in focus, where people can make a living supplying services to those in need (Kolsky & Diop, 2004). Economic aspects are further discussed in chapter 9 and in relation to institutional and legal aspects in chapter 10.

1.4.4 Sociocultural aspects and use

Sociocultural factors are fundamental for sustainability. A sanitation facility without appeal will not be used. Use is linked to access and convenience factors, but is also governed by social, cultural and religious beliefs. For girls and women, safe access is a major concern. The perception of ownership or responsibility is crucial and will affect, for example, the cleanliness of the facilities and, ultimately, their long-term success. Sociocultural issues concerning the use of excreta and greywater are further discussed in chapter 7.

1.4.5 Technology function

Technology function and selection contribute importantly to aspects of sustainability. Technologies selected for the safe use of excreta and greywater should meet all of the following sustainability criteria, accounting for robustness and variabilities in load:

- Health – technologies should provide inherent individual and public health protection;
- Environment – technologies should prevent contaminants from reaching groundwater and surface water supplies and provide other environmental protection;
- Economy – technologies should be cost-effective and available in a range of options that accommodate different levels of affordability, and it should be possible to upgrade or improve them as more resources become available;
- Sociocultural – technologies should be compatible with local values and beliefs and designed with all potential users in mind.

Excreta and greywater treatment technologies, handling and use are further discussed in chapter 5.

1.5 Driving forces

Driving forces behind the increased use of excreta and greywater in agriculture worldwide include:

- increasing water scarcity and stress, and degradation of freshwater resources resulting from improper disposal of excreta and greywater;
- population increase and related increased demand for food and fibre;
- a growing recognition of the resource value of excreta and greywater and the nutrients they contain;
- the MDGs, especially the goals for ensuring environmental sustainability and for eliminating poverty and hunger.

1.5.1 Water scarcity, stress and degradation

It is estimated that within the next 50 years, more than 40% of the world's population will live in countries facing water stress or water scarcity. In 1995, 31 countries were classified as water-scarce or water-stressed, and it is estimated that 48 and 54 countries will fall into these categories by 2025 and 2050, respectively. These numbers do not include people living in arid regions of large countries where sufficient water is poorly distributed — e.g. China, India and the United States of America (China is predicted to reach water scarcity by 2050 and India by 2025) (Hinrichsen, Robey & Upadhyay, 1998). Growing competition between agricultural and urban areas for high-quality freshwater supplies, particularly in arid, semi-arid and densely populated regions, will increase the pressure on this resource.

Excreta and greywater can be treated and used close to their origin, either on site or in decentralized treatment systems. This prevents their discharge into surface waters, thus reducing downstream microbial and chemical contamination. It also reduces the costs of developing infrastructure for elaborate conveyance systems (e.g. sewer networks).

Additionally, the "polluter pays" principle is starting to take hold in many places, forcing upstream users to treat their wastes to higher standards before discharging them into water bodies. Previously, the additional costs of water treatment or loss of ecosystem services (e.g. destruction of fisheries or loss of aesthetic value) were passed on to downstream water users. Acknowledgement of the concept of integrated water resources management has led to the realization that waste discharges into surface waters have health, environmental and economic implications for downstream users. As this awareness spreads, it will become increasingly difficult to discharge inadequately treated wastes into surface waters. Therefore, treatment and use of excreta and greywater closer to the point at which they are generated become a more attractive option.

1.5.2 Population growth and food production

Over the next 50 years, most population growth is expected to occur in urban and periurban areas in developing countries (United Nations Population Division, 2002). For example, a majority of the 19 cities for which the most rapid growth is predicted between 2000 and 2015 (with populations expected to more than double) are in chronically water-short regions of the developing world (United Nations Population Division, 2002).

The growth of urban populations, especially in developing countries, will lead to several new challenges:

- greater populations will generate more wastes, especially in and around cities;
- on-site waste disposal will be more difficult in many densely populated areas;
- urban agriculture will play a more important role in supplying food to city dwellers. Excreta and greywater will become increasingly important as inputs.

Excreta and greywater can help to improve food production, especially for subsistence farmers who otherwise might not be able to afford artificial fertilizers. The use of greywater for irrigating home gardens may also help to relieve malnutrition and food insecurity at the household level by providing a steady supply of water for crop irrigation, allowing the year-long production of vegetables.

The use of treated and source-separated faeces and urine has been suggested as suitable for urban agriculture. Wastewater is used already to a large extent in these applications. Treated excreta would potentially pose fewer health risks in these types of applications. Esrey (2001) has summarized the impact of excreta use in relation to nutrients in urban areas.

Eighty per cent of the world's natural food resources are converted into waste and disposed of (Smit, 2000). According to predictions for 2015, about 26 cities in the world are expected to have a population of over 10 million people, which implies the need to import an estimated 6000 tonnes of food each day (FAO, 1998). More than 50% of the absolute poor live in urban areas and spend much of their income on food. Their dietary intakes are nutrient limited, and urban residents in developing countries have a lower energy intake than their rural counterparts. Yet poor urban dwellers will not be able to afford imported food.

Lowering the costs of inputs and producing food closer to where people live can reduce food production costs. Urban agriculture and home gardening can produce more food per unit space, because food can be grown on roofs, on walls and in and around buildings. Urban agriculture has enjoyed a revival in the past few decades (Smit, Ratta & Nasr, 1996). In greater Bangkok, 60% of the land is under cultivation. The demand for food by consumers and for water and nutrients by producers reconnects resources and wastes in a safe, non-polluting and economic fashion. Growing food closer to consumers also strengthens the livelihood of local communities.

Recovery and recycling of nutrients from human excreta and other organic matter provide complete nutrition for plants. Access to affordable and more nutritious food will increase and post-harvest food losses will be reduced if food is grown and consumed locally. This represents a saving in water as well as nutrients.

When food is grown farther away from population centres, not only does it cost more, but valuable micronutrients are less likely to reach consumers, particularly people with little income. Urban farming and home gardening, on the other hand, can result in better diets, improving macro- and micronutrient intakes as well as the nutritional status of vulnerable groups, such as women, children, the elderly and the disabled (Maxwell, Levin & Csete, 1998).

1.5.3 Excreta and greywater as resources

Excreta and greywater contain nutrients and water, which make them valuable resources. The use of excreta and greywater in agriculture, aquaculture and other settings reduces the need for artificial fertilizers and is important for nutrient recycling. Some studies indicate that the world's supply of readily available phosphorus is limited and will run out in 150 years (Rosemarin, 2004). Excreta are an accessible source of important plant nutrients, such as phosphorus, nitrogen and potassium. Excreta use can help to reduce the mining of finite phosphorus reserves and energy expended to create artificial fertilizers. Greywater is mostly used for irrigation, as service water or sometimes for groundwater recharge at a local scale. Its use helps reduce the demand for freshwater supply and mitigates the stress on water resources.

Excreta quantities and composition

Annually, about 130 million tonnes of fertilizers are sold globally, 63% of which are sold in the developing world. Of this quantity, 78 million tonnes are nitrogen and 13.7 million tonnes phosphorus. The rest represents potassium, sulfur and micronutrients. The excreta from 6 billion persons contain 27 million tonnes of nitrogen and 3 million tonnes of phosphorus. This means that one third of the world's mineral nitrogen use could in theory be replaced by nitrogen from excreta. Similarly, 22% of the world's use of mined phosphorus could be replaced by phosphorus from excreta.

The major plant nutrients nitrogen, phosphorus and potassium are found in human excreta and thus also in domestic wastewater (Figure 1.2), but the contents will vary depending on the food intake. Greywater will mainly recycle water and supplies only minor amounts of nutrients.

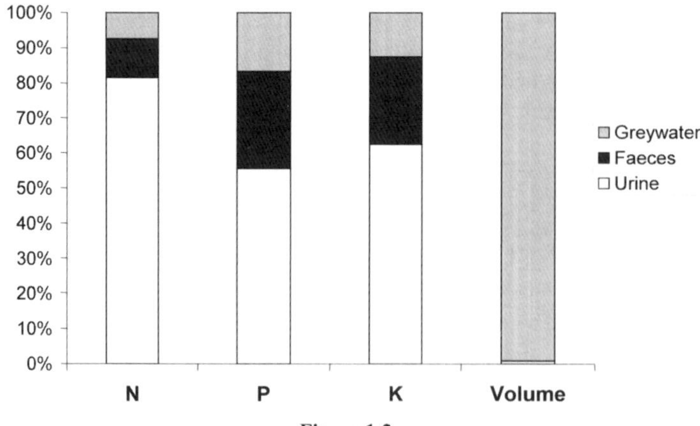

Figure 1.2

Content of major plant nutrients and volume in domestic wastewater in Sweden. The daily mean excretion per person and per day is 13 g nitrogen (N), 1.5 g phosphorus (P) and 4 g potassium (K) in a volume of 150–200 litres, including greywater (Vinnerås, 2002).

Mass balance and content of macronutrients in excreta

The nutrient content in urine and faeces depends directly on the amounts and quality of food consumed. Children need nutrients to grow; in adults, however, food consumption is mainly for energy, and only minor amounts of nutrients are retained and accumulated in the body. Almost all consumed plant nutrients will therefore leave the human body in excreta. Even during adolescence, accumulation of nutrients in the body is negligible, calculated to be less than 2% of the consumed nitrogen between the ages of 3 and 13.

Since most nutrients leave the human body in excreta, excreted plant nutrients can be calculated from food intake, on which information is readily available. Based on statistics from the Food and Agriculture Organization of the United Nations (FAO) (http://www.fao.org) on the available food supply in different countries, calculations have been made of amounts and macronutrient content of excreta (Jönsson & Vinnerås, 2004). Table 1.1 provides default values for these parameters in Sweden.

Table 1.1 Swedish default values for excreted mass and nutrients

Parameter	Unit	Urine	Faeces	Toilet paper	Blackwater (urine + faeces)
Wet mass	kg/person per year	550	51	8.9	610
Dry mass	kg/person per year	21	11	8.5	40.5
Nitrogen	g/person per year	4000	550		4550
Phosphorus	g/person per year	365	183		548

Source: Vinnerås (2002).

The estimated average amounts of excreta, food intake (according to FAO statistics) and nutrient content in different foodstuffs are used in a relationship (Equations 1 and 2) between food intake (according to FAO) and the excretion of nitrogen and phosphorus:

$$N = 0.13 \times \text{total food protein} \qquad \textbf{Equation 1}$$

$$P = 0.011 \times (\text{total food protein} + \text{vegetal food protein}) \qquad \textbf{Equation 2}$$

These equations can be used to estimate the average excretion of nitrogen and phosphorus in different countries; see examples in Table 1.2. There tends to be greater variability in values for potassium.

The total per capita annual excretion reported by Gao et al. (2002) for China was 4.4 kg of nitrogen and 0.5 kg of phosphorus, which are in the same range as the figures given in Table 1.2, where the total excretion has been partitioned between urine and faeces.

The relative amounts of nutrients in urine and faeces depend on the diet: digested nutrients are mainly excreted with the urine, whereas undigested fractions are excreted in the faeces. Approximately 88% of the excreta nitrogen and 67% of the excreta phosphorus are found in the urine, and the rest are in the faeces. These figures are lower in China, where the urine contains approximately 70% of the excreta nitrogen and 25–60% of the phosphorus (Gao et al., 2002).

Digestibility also influences the amount of faeces excreted. In Sweden, the amount of faeces excreted is estimated at 51 kg wet mass/person per year (11 kg dry weight) (Vinnerås, 2002). In China, faecal excretion is estimated at 115 kg wet mass/person per year (22 kg dry weight) (Gao et al., 2002).

Table 1.2 Estimated excretion of nutrients per capita in different countries

Country		Excretion rate (kg/person per year)		
		Nitrogen	Phosphorus	Potassium
China, total		4.0	0.6	1.8
	Urine	3.5	0.4	1.3
	Faeces	0.5	0.2	0.5
Haiti, total		2.1	0.3	1.2
	Urine	1.9	0.2	0.9
	Faeces	0.3	0.1	0.3
India, total		2.7	0.4	1.5
	Urine	2.3	0.3	1.1
	Faeces	0.3	0.1	0.4
South Africa, total		3.4	0.5	1.6
	Urine	3.0	0.3	1.2
	Faeces	0.4	0.2	0.4
Uganda, total		2.5	0.4	1.4
	Urine	2.2	0.3	1.0
	Faeces	0.3	0.1	0.4

Source: Jönsson & Vinnerås (2004).

The concentration of nutrients in the excreted urine depends on the nutrients and liquid intake, level of personal activity and climate conditions. The liquid intake is in the range of 0.8–1.5 litres per person per day (up to 550 litres per person per year) for adults and about half that amount for children in Europe (Lentner, Lentner & Wink, 1981), but it may be much higher due to climate or activity level. Similar amounts have been reported for China: 1.6 litres per person per day (580 litres per person per year) (Gao et al., 2002). Excessive perspiration results in concentrated urine, while consumption of large amounts of liquid dilutes the urine.

Use of urine as fertilizer

Urine is rich in nitrogen and can be used for fertilizing most non-nitrogen-fixing crops after proper treatment to reduce potential microbial contamination. Crops with a high nitrogen content that respond well to nitrogen fertilization include spinach, cauliflower and maize. Direct use of urine as a plant fertilizer will entail the most efficient use of nutrients, but addition of urine to improve composting of carbon-rich substrates is another possibility (although it may result in large ammonia losses). The nutrients in urine are in ionic form, and their plant availability and fertilizing effect compare well with those of chemical (ammonium- and urea-based) fertilizers (Kirchmann & Petterson, 1995; Johansson et al., 2001). When the nitrogen content of collected urine is unknown, a concentration of 3–7 g of nitrogen per litre at excretion can be used as a default value (Jönsson & Vinnerås, 2004). On a yearly basis, the amount of nitrogen produced per person equals 30–70 kg, supporting one crop on 300–400 m^2, but up to 3–4 times this level may be an optimal application strategy.

The achieved yield varies depending on the soil conditions. As with chemical fertilizers, the effect is lower on soil poor in organic content. Under these conditions, soil fertility may benefit from using both urine and faeces or other organic fertilizers alternatively applied in consecutive years and for different crops. Urine can be applied either undiluted or diluted with water, preferentially just before sowing or during the initial plant growth. Once the crop enters its reproductive stage, nutrient uptake is low, and nutrients are mainly relocated within the plant (Marschner, 1997). Plants with inefficient or small root systems (e.g. carrots, onions and lettuce) will benefit from repeated applications during the cultivation period (Thorup-Kristensen, 2001). The test results of the use of urine as a fertilizer for barley in Sweden are shown in Box 1.1.

The best fertilizing effect is obtained when the urine is directly incorporated into the soil after application; shallow incorporation is sufficient (Rodhe, Richert Stintzing & Steineck, 2004). Direct incorporation also minimizes ammonia losses to the air. Surface application generally gives a nitrogen loss above 70% due to ammonia volatilization, and soil incorporation is therefore very important (Morken, 1998).

Trials with different application strategies using urine as a fertilizer for leeks gave a threefold yield increase (Båth, 2003). Application either in two doses or divided into smaller doses applied every 14 days gave the same yield and nutrient uptake (Table 1.3). The strategy used in West Africa involves the frequent application of small amounts of urine in order to avoid leaching. Extensive trials have been performed on various vegetables in Zimbabwe (Morgan, 2004). Results confirm the experience that urine is a quick-acting fertilizer that can be used for most vegetables.

Table 1.3 Results of a field trial using human urine as a fertilizer for leeks

Treatment[a]		Nitrogen application rate (kg/ha)[b]	Yield (t/ha)[b]	Nitrogen yield (kg/ha)[b]
A	Urine every 14 days	150	54	111
B	Urine twice	150	51	110
C	Urine every 14 days + extra potassium	150	55	115
D	Unfertilized	0	17	24

[a] No statistically significant difference between treatments A, B and C.
[b] kg/ha = g/10 m^2; t/ha = kg/10 m^2.
Source: After Båth (2003).

Use of faeces as fertilizer

Faeces may contain high concentrations of pathogens, and appropriate treatment is therefore crucial to ensure its safe use. The total amount of nutrients excreted is lower in faeces than in urine, but the concentrations of (especially) phosphorus and potassium are higher in faeces than in urine. It is these two elements that may significantly increase the crop yield (Morgan, 2003). The content of organic matter in faeces also increases the water-holding and ion-buffering capacities of soils, which is of importance for improving soil structure and stimulates the microbial activity. The fertilizing effect of faeces is more variable than that of urine, since the proportion of nitrogen in mineral form and the content and properties of the organic matter vary depending on the treatment applied.

Faecal compost applied together with urine may have advantages, since the former conditions the soil and the latter provides rapidly accessible nitrogen. Incineration of faeces results in ash with high contents of phosphorus and potassium as well as micronutrients, but nitrogen and sulfur are lost to the atmosphere. Ash in general (which may also be added to the faeces) also increases the pH and the buffering capacity of the soil. The pH increase is especially important on soils with very low pH (4–5) and to get the full benefit from fertilizing with, for example, urine, as shown on experimental plots in Zimbabwe (Morgan, 2005).

Box 1.1 Urine as fertilizer for barley in Sweden

Urine was tested as a fertilizer on barley in Sweden during 1997–1999 (Johansson et al., 2001; Rodhe, Richert Stintzing & Steineck, 2004). Results showed that the nitrogen effect of urine corresponded to about 90% of that of equal amounts of ammonium nitrate mineral fertilizers (Figure 1.3). The urine was spread before sowing with a conventional spreader for liquid manure (Figure 1.4).

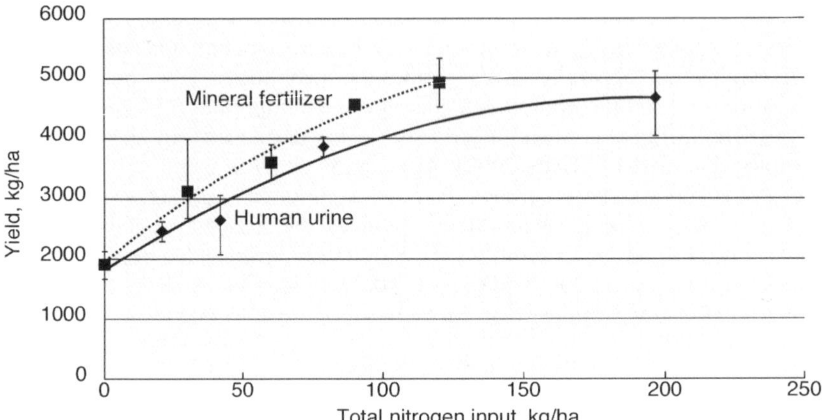

Figure 1.3
Results from field trials with urine as fertilizer for barley, 1999

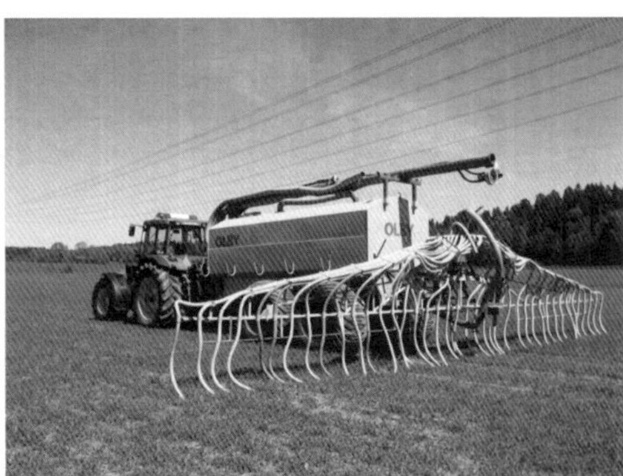

Figure 1.4
Conventional slurry spreader used for application of urine

Faecal compost can be applied as a complete phosphorus–potassium fertilizer or as a soil improver. Approximately 40–70% of the organic matter and somewhat less of the nitrogen are lost through biological activity and volatilization. Most of the remaining nitrogen will become available to plants during degradation. This slow process improves the water-holding and buffering capacity of the soil. The phosphorus is also partly, but to a lesser extent, bound in organic forms, whereas the potassium is mainly in ionic form and readily available to plants. In anaerobic digests, approximately the same proportion of organic matter is degraded as in composting, but the mineralized nitrogen remains within the digested residue and 40–70% of the nitrogen is in the form of ammonium, which is readily available to plants. The digested residues make up a well balanced, quick-acting and complete fertilizer (Åkerhielm & Richert Stintzing, 2004). Additional substrates, such as animal manure and household waste, are often added to digestion processes, which affects the amount and composition of the residue.

If faeces are dried rapidly and low moisture levels prevail, the loss of organic matter and nitrogen will be small. Compared with composting, dry storage recycles more organic matter and nitrogen to the soil, but the organic matter is less stable. Dried faecal matter is a complete phosphorus–potassium fertilizer, contributing considerable amounts of nitrogen as well.

Treated faeces, in a desiccated, incinerated, composted or mixed form, is preferably applied to and incorporated in the root zone of the soil prior to sowing or planting, because the high content and availability of phosphorus are important for the development of small plants and roots.

The faecal matter from one person is enough to fertilize 200–300 m^2 of wheat at a yield of 3000 kg/ha based on the P content. Where the soil is devoid of phosphorus, 5–10 times the removal rate can be applied. At this application rate, most of the phosphorus will remain and will improve the soil, with significant yield increases and without negative effects from phosphorus or organic matter. Application rates for farmyard manure in agriculture are in the range of 20–40 t/ha. If large amounts of lime or ash are used as additives, a minor risk of negative effects exists at high application rates, due to a high resulting pH (>7.5–8) in the soil. This risk will, however, materialize only at extremely high application rates or if the initial pH of the soil is already high.

In bucket experiments of low-temperature composting of faeces in Zimbabwe, vegetables such as spinach, covo, lettuce, green pepper, tomato and onion were grown in 10-litre buckets with poor local topsoil (Morgan, 2003). Growth was compared between no additions and plants grown in topsoil mixed with an equal volume of humus derived from co-composted human faeces and urine. A dramatic increase in vegetable yield resulted from the addition of the composted faeces and urine mix to poor soil (Table 1.4).

Table 1.4 Average yields in plant trials comparing growth in topsoil only with growth in a mixture consisting of 50% topsoil and 50% Fossa alterna compost

Plant and soil type	Growth period	Yield (g fresh weight) in topsoil only	Yield (g fresh weight) in 50/50 topsoil/Fossa alterna soil	Relative yield improvement rate
Spinach, Epworth soil (*n* = 6)	30 days	72	546	7.6
Covo, Epworth soil (*n* = 3)	30 days	20	161	8.1
Covo 2, Epworth soil (*n* = 6)	30 days	81	357	4.4
Lettuce, Epworth soil (*n* = 6)	30 days	122	912	7.5
Onion, Ruwa soil (*n* = 9)	4 months	141	391	2.8
Green pepper, Ruwa soil (*n* = 1)	4 months	19	89	4.7
Tomato, Ruwa soil	3 months	73	735	10.1

Source: Morgan (2003).

Greywater volume and composition

Greywater production and composition are dependent on sanitary standards, awareness of the need for water conservation, water availability and raw water composition (Lens, Zeeman & Lettinga, 2001; Eriksson et al., 2002). Greywater volume and composition also vary with lifestyle: family size, age of residents, eating habits and detergents used. The main sources of greywater are laundry, bathroom and kitchen. In the following summary, the results of some studies on greywater volume and composition are presented.

Greywater volumes produced may be as low as 20–30 litres per person per day in poor areas where water often is hand-carried from taps (Ridderstolpe, 2004; Winblad & Simpson-Hébert, 2004). When availability increases, the production of greywater increases, but it seldom exceeds 100 litres per person per day in developing countries. In industrialized countries, greywater production is normally in the range of 100–200 litres per person per day (the highest figures are reported from the USA and Canada) and sometimes exceeds 200 litres per person per day (Crites & Tchobanoglous, 1998; Bertaglial et al., 2005). In new housing developments in Europe, where awareness of the need for water conservation is promoted, the per capita daily greywater production is less than 100 litres (Table 1.5).

In general, the concentrations of plant nutrients (nitrogen, phosphorus and potassium) and pathogens of health concern are low in greywater (Ottosson & Stenström, 2003a; Jenssen & Vråle, 2004), due to the fact that the majority of these are found in excreta. Bacterial indicators tend to overestimate the faecal load in greywater because regrowth may occur (Manville et al., 2001); compared with chemical biomarkers, a 100- to 1000-fold overestimation of the faecal load was found (Ottosson & Stenström, 2003a). The microbial contamination of greywater is, however, significant and must be taken into account when calculating risks and selecting treatment methods.

Table 1.5 Examples of greywater production

Location	Greywater production (litres per person per day)	Reference
China, ecological sanitation project	80	EcoSanRes (2005b)
Belgium	85	Bertaglial et al. (2005)
Germany	35–65	Panesar & Lange (2001)
Germany, Eco-village Flintenbreite	60	Ridderstolpe (2004)
Germany, Norway and Sweden, new built house area, water conservation	<100	Ridderstolpe (2004); Winblad & Simpson-Hébert (2004)
Norway, ecovillage	81	Kristiansen & Skaarer (1979)
Norway, student dormitories, water conservation	112	Jenssen (2001)
Sweden, range for ecovillages	66–110	Vinnerås et al. (2006)
Sweden, proposed norm	100	Vinnerås et al. (2006)
Sweden, existing norm	150	Vinnerås et al. (2006)
Europe, northern part	110	Lens, Zeeman & Lettinga (2001)
Australia, western part	112	Department of Health (2002)
USA	200	Crites & Tchobanoglous (1998); Bertaglial et al. (2005)
Developing regions	20–30	Ridderstolpe (2004); Winblad & Simpson-Hébert (2004)
Range	70–275	Otterpohl (2002)

Greywater contributes 10–30% of the total phosphorus input to a combined wastewater system, and the concentrations are governed by the type of detergents (Rasmussen, Jenssen & Westlie, 1996; Vinnerås, 2002; Jenssen & Vråle, 2004). If phosphorus-containing detergents are used, concentrations typically range from 3 to 7 mg/l. If phosphate-free detergents are used, the concentrations are about 1 mg/l. Greywater contributes 10% or less of the total nitrogen content in wastewater, and the nitrogen concentration in greywater is often 10 mg/l or less, prior to treatment (Vinnerås, 2002; Jenssen & Vråle, 2004).

Greywater contains 50% or more of the readily degradable organic matter in household sewage — measured as biological (BOD) or chemical (COD) oxygen demand — but the concentrations are highly variable, depending on household practices. In industrialized countries, excessive amounts of detergents, including shampoos, shower oils, cleansing powders, etc., are common and responsible for substantial BOD input, in addition to grease and oil used in food preparation. In cultures where use of cooking oil is common, the greywater organic content becomes very high and may call for special care when designing treatment systems. If collected separately, the oil and grease can be processed to biodiesel (Zhang et al., 2003), but they can also increase biogas yield in anaerobic digestion. Examples of concentrations of various water quality parameters found in untreated or primary treated greywater are presented in Table 1.6.

The concentrations of nutrients in greywater depend on the per capita mass discharge and the water use. The per capita discharges under Swedish conditions are presented in Table 1.7.

In the sites listed in Table 1.7, phosphorus-containing detergents were used. According to Norwegian studies, the per capita mass discharge of phosphorus is reduced to 0.2 mg/l with phosphorus-free detergents (Jenssen & Vråle, 2004). The major part of the heavy metal load in household wastewater is found in the greywater fraction (Vinnerås, 2002), and concentrations of heavy metals can therefore be expected to be on the same level as in combined household wastewater.

1.5.4 Millennium Development Goals

At the 2002 World Summit on Sustainable Development in Johannesburg, global leaders agreed to adopt a sanitation coverage target — namely, "to halve, by the year 2015, the proportion of people who do not have access to basic sanitation" (United Nations, 2002). Expanding access to and proper use of improved sanitation facilities would have far-ranging positive health consequences and would support meeting the relevant targets of the Millennium Development Goals.

To achieve the sanitation target under MDG7, WHO estimates that 1.9 billion people will need to gain access to improved sanitation by 2015 — 1 billion urban dwellers and 900 million rural dwellers. This figure takes into account the projected population growth. As of 2002, 77% of the unserved worldwide (i.e. 2 billion people) lived in rural areas. Expanding access to basic sanitation in rural areas is an urgent priority (WHO/UNICEF, 2004). A large percentage of population growth, however, is expected to occur in urban and periurban areas (often in slums or informal settlements) in developing countries.

Many of the 2.6 billion people without improved sanitation are among those hardest to reach: families living in remote rural areas and urban slums, families displaced by war and famine and families mired in the poverty/disease trap (WHO/UNICEF, 2004).

Table 1.6 Concentrations of some water quality parameters found in untreated or primary treated (septic tank effluent) greywater

Country/reference	Parameters							
	BOD_5 (mg/l)	COD (mg/l)	Suspended solids (mg/l)	Total N (mg/l)	NH_4 (mg/l)	Kjeldahl N (mg/l)	Total P (mg/l)	Faecal coliforms (log numbers/ 100 ml)
Canada / Brandes (1978)	149	366	162	11.5	1.7	11.3	1.4[a]	6.2
Norway / Kristiansen & Skaarer (1979)	130	341	35	19	11.5		1.3 (0.42[b])	5.1
USA[c] / Siegrist & Boyle (1981)	178	456	45			15.9	4.4	6.2
Sweden norm / Naturvårds-verket (1995)	187		107	6.7			4 (1.0[b])	
Norway[c] / Rasmussen, Jenssen & Westlie (1996)	116		39	42.2	36.1		3.97	
Australia / Department of Health (2002)	160		115		5.3	12	8	5.2
Norway[c] / Jenssen (2001)	88	277	–	8.8	3.8	4.9	1.0[b]	4–6
Sweden proposed norm / Vinnerås et al. (2006)	260[c]	520		13.6			5.2	
Germany / Li et al. (2004)	73–142			8.7–13.1	2.5		6.8–9.2	4–6
Malaysia[d] / Jenssen et al. (2005)	128	212	75	37	12.6	22.2	2.4	5.8

BOD_5, five-day biological oxygen demand

[a] Excluding laundry.

[b] Phosphorus-free detergents.

[c] BOD_7, seven-day biological oxygen demand, for the Swedish proposed norm.

[d] Septic tank effluent.

In urban and periurban centres, much of the sanitation expansion may be in the form of sewerage (conventional sewerage in urban centres and simplified sewerage in periurban areas or slums). Sewerage systems are expensive to build and maintain and require relatively large volumes of water to function properly (simplified sewerage systems require less water than full sewerage systems). Although sewer systems protect the health of the user, health gains may be limited for the community as a whole, because much of the wastewater is likely to be discharged into water bodies without adequate treatment, thus exposing downstream users to human pathogens through untreated drinking-water, food or contact with contaminated water.

Table 1.7 Greywater volume and concentrations of various water quality parameters in greywater collected from Swedish eco-housing developments compared with Swedish norm values

Parameters	Ekoporten	Gebers	Vibyåsen	Swedish norm	Proposed norm
Volume (litres per person per day)	104	110	66	150	100.0
Dry mass (g/person per day)	59.2	15.1	29.2	20	59.8
BOD_7 (g/person per day)		21.1	27.7	28.0	26.0
COD (g/person per day)		47.9	39.0	72.0	52.1
Nitrogen (g/person per day)	1.7	1.4	0.6	1.0	1.4
Phosphorus (g/person per day)	0.4	0.6	0.5	0.3	0.5
Potassium (g/person per day)	4.0	1.0	0.5	0.5	1.0

BOD_7, seven-day biological oxygen demand

Source: Calculated from Vinnerås et al. (2006).

Therefore, if effective treatment were available at the household level, prior to discharge of waste into the environment or use, the health of downstream users would be better protected.

Poverty has long been recognized as one of the primary impediments to sustainable development. In many countries, poor subsistence farmers do not have access to water resources and may not have money to buy fertilizers. The use of excreta and greywater in agriculture has the potential to affect poverty positively in several ways:

- improved household food security and nutritional variety, which reduce malnutrition;
- increased income from sale of surplus crops (the use of excreta and greywater may allow cultivation of crops year-round in some locations);
- money saved on fertilizer, which can be put to other productive uses.

However, increased poverty may also result when poor management and dangerous practices lead to negative public health outcomes.

The use of excreta and greywater in agriculture is therefore a key development issue and is at the centre of the sanitation debate. Poor households spend a larger percentage (50–80%) of their income on food and water than do households that are better off (Lipton, 1983; World Food Programme, 1995). Without access to resources such as excreta or greywater, many poor families would not be able to meet their nutritional needs or would spend more money on food and less on other health-promoting activities, such as primary health care or education.

2 THE STOCKHOLM FRAMEWORK

The Stockholm Framework is an integrated approach that combines risk assessment and risk management to control water-related diseases. It was developed for infectious diseases, but it can be equally applied to diseases resulting from exposures to toxic chemicals. This chapter contains a summary of the components of the Stockholm Framework and how it applies to assessing and managing risk associated with the use of excreta and greywater in agriculture. Applied management and monitoring are discussed in more detail in chapters 5 and 6.

2.1 A harmonized approach to risk assessment/management

Following an expert meeting in Stockholm, Sweden, WHO published *Water quality — Guidelines, standards and health: Assessment of risk and risk management for water-related infectious disease* (Fewtrell & Bartram, 2001). This report provides a harmonized framework for the development of health-based guidelines and standards for water- and sanitation-related microbial hazards. The Stockholm Framework involves the assessment of health risks prior to the setting of health-based targets and the development of guideline values, defining basic control approaches and evaluating the impact of these combined approaches on public health.

The Framework encourages countries to adjust guidelines to local social, cultural, economic and environmental circumstances and compare the health risks associated with, for example, excreta and greywater use in agriculture with risks from microbial exposures through other routes, such as food, hygiene practices, drinking-water or recreational/occupational water contact. This approach aims to facilitate the management of infectious diseases in an integrated, holistic fashion, not in isolation from other diseases or exposure pathways. Disease outcomes from different exposure routes can be compared by using a common metric, such as disability adjusted life years (DALYs), or normalized for a population over a time period (see Box 2.1).

Box 2.1 Disability adjusted life years (DALYs)

DALYs are a measure of the health of a population or burden of disease due to a specific disease or risk factor. DALYs attempt to measure the time lost because of disability or death from a disease compared with a long life free of disability in the absence of the disease. DALYs are calculated by adding the years of life lost to premature death to the years lived with a disability. Years of life lost are calculated from age-specific mortality rates and the standard life expectancies of a given population. Years lived with a disability are calculated from the number of cases multiplied by the average duration of the disease and a severity factor ranging from 1 (death) to 0 (perfect health) based on the disease (e.g. watery diarrhoea has a severity factor ranging from 0.09 to 0.12, depending on the age group) (Murray & Lopez, 1996; Prüss & Havelaar, 2001). DALYs are an important tool for comparing health outcomes, because they account not only for acute health effects but also for delayed and chronic effects — including morbidity and mortality (Bartram, Fewtrell & Stenström, 2001).

When risk is described in DALYs, different health outcomes (e.g. cancer vs giardiasis) can be compared and risk management decisions can be prioritized.

WHO water- and sanitation-related guidelines have been developed in accordance with the principles of the Stockholm Framework. The third edition of the WHO *Guidelines for drinking-water quality* (WHO, 2004a) and the WHO *Guidelines for safe recreational water environments* (WHO, 2003a, 2005a) have both incorporated a harmonized approach to risk assessment and management as outlined in the Stockholm Framework.

2.2 Elements of the Stockholm Framework

The individual elements of the Stockholm Framework and how they specifically relate to the use of excreta and greywater are presented in Figure 2.1 and in Table 2.1. Some of the Framework elements are discussed in more detail in subsequent chapters of this document.

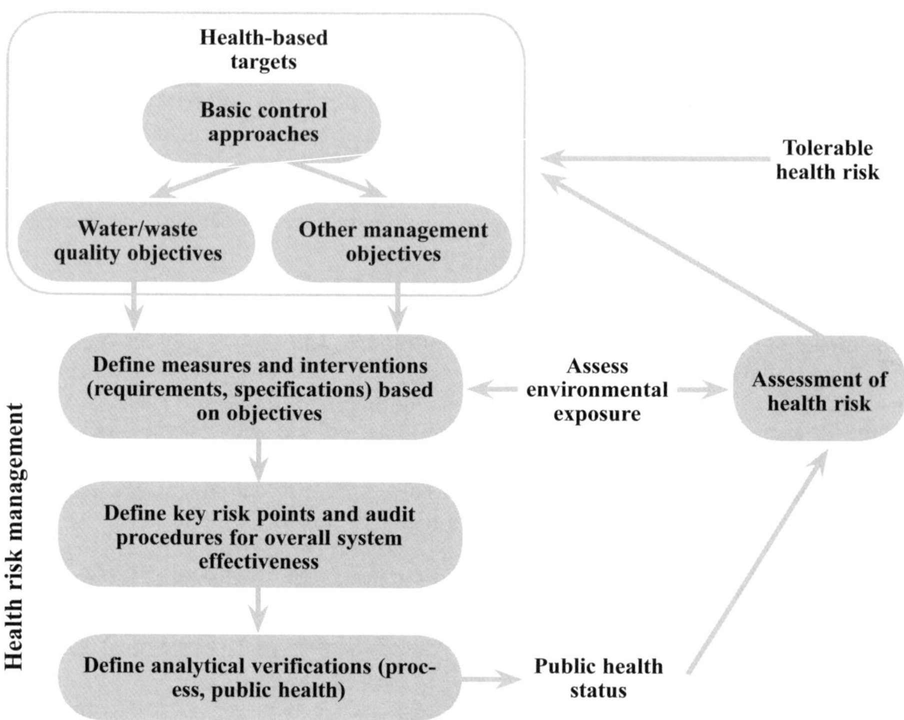

Figure 2.1
The Stockholm Framework for developing harmonized guidelines for the management of water-related infectious disease (adapted from Bartram, Fewtrell & Stenström 2001)

Table 2.1 Elements and important considerations of the Stockholm Framework

Framework component	Process	Considerations
Assessment of health risk	Epidemiological studies	Best estimate of risk — not overly conservative
		Health outcomes presented in DALYs facilitate comparison of risks across different exposures and priority setting
	QMRA	Assessment of risk is an iterative process — risk should be periodically reassessed based on new data or changing conditions
		Risk assessment (QMRA) is a tool for estimating risk and should be supported by other data (e.g. outbreak investigations, epidemiological evidence and studies of environmental behaviour of microbes)
		Process dependent on quality of data
		Risk assessment needs to account for short-term underperformance

Table 2.1 (continued)

Framework component	Process	Considerations
Tolerable risk/health-based targets	Health-based target setting linked to risk assessment	Needs to be realistic and achievable within the constraints of each setting Set based on a risk–benefit approach; should consider cost-effectiveness of different available interventions Should take sensitive subpopulations into account Reference pathogens should be selected for relevance to contamination, control challenges and health significance (it may be necessary to select more than one reference pathogen) Health-based targets establish a desired health outcome
Health risk management	Define water/waste quality objectives Define other management objectives Define measures and interventions Define key risk points and audit procedures Define analytical verifications	Health-based targets should be basis for selecting risk management strategies; can combine exposure prevention through good practices and appropriate water quality objectives Risk points should be defined and used to anticipate and minimize health risks; parameters for monitoring can be set up around risk points A multiple-barrier approach should be used Monitoring — overall emphasis should be given to periodic inspection/auditing and to simple measurements that can be rapidly and frequently made to inform management Risk management strategies need to address rare or catastrophic events Analytical verifications may include testing wastewater and/or crops for *E. coli* or viable helminth eggs to confirm that the treatment processes are working to the desired level Validation of the effectiveness of the health protection measures is needed to ensure that the system is capable of meeting the health-based targets; validation is needed when a new system is developed or additional barriers are added; information should be used to make adjustments to the risk management process to improve safety
Public health status	Public health surveillance	Need to evaluate effectiveness of risk management interventions on specific health outcomes (through both investigation of disease outbreaks and evaluation of background disease levels) Public health outcome monitoring provides the information needed to fine-tune risk management process through an iterative process; procedures for estimating the burden of disease will facilitate monitoring health outcomes due to specific exposures Burden of disease estimates can be used to place water-related exposures in the wider public health context to enable prioritization of risk management decisions

Source: Adapted from Carr & Bartram (2004).

2.3 Assessment of environmental exposure

The assessment of environmental exposure is an important input to both risk assessment and risk management. It is a process that looks at the hazards in the environment and evaluates different routes of exposure for human (or animal) populations.

The primary hazard is related to exposure to pathogens in untreated or insufficiently treated faecal excreta transmitted through the faecal–oral route. Excreted urine may also contain pathogens, but to a lesser extent and in a lesser range of etiological agents (see chapter 3). The excreta may contaminate food or water. Several helminths in excreta may also infect humans through the skin. Direct contact with contaminated material and subsequent accidental ingestion from contaminated fingers or utensils are a major transmission pathway. Contact may occur before treatment, during treatment, including handling, or when the material is used/applied to soil. Additionally, contamination of foods may occur directly from use, but also through unhygienic practices in the kitchen. Even if the fertilized crop is to be cooked before consumption, surfaces may be contaminated and pathogens transferred to other foods or fluids.

2.4 Assessment of health risk

Risk is the likelihood that something with a negative impact will occur. The agent that causes the adverse effect is a *hazard.* Risk incorporates the probability that an event will occur with the effect that it will have on a population or the environment, accounting for the sociopolitical context where it takes place (Cutter, 1993).

The assessment of risks is central in preventive public health. It can be carried out directly via epidemiological studies or indirectly through quantitative microbial risk assessment (QMRA).

Epidemiological studies aim to assess the health risks by comparing the level of disease in the exposed population (e.g. a population using excreta/greywater in agriculture or consuming products grown with them) with that in an unexposed or control population. The difference in disease levels may then be attributed to the practice of using the excreta/greywater, provided that the two populations compared are similar in all other respects, including socioeconomic status and ethnicity. Potential confounding factors and bias, which could affect results, need to be addressed. There have been very few epidemiological studies concerned with the use of excreta or greywater in agriculture. Blumenthal & Peasey (2002) review some (see also chapter 3).

The indirect assessment of risk in QMRA is usually dealt with in a step-wise approach. *Risk analysis* embraces the three components of risk assessment (i.e. QMRA), risk management and risk communication (Haas, Rose & Gerba, 1999). *Risk assessment* is the qualitative or quantitative characterization and estimation of potential adverse health effects associated with exposure of individuals or populations to hazards (i.e. microbial agents). *Risk management* is the process of controlling risks, weighing alternatives and selecting appropriate action, accounting for values, engineering, economics and legal and political issues. *Risk communication* is the communication of risks to managers, stakeholders, public officials and the public. It includes public perception and the ability to exchange information.

QMRA can be used as a predictive tool to indirectly estimate the risk to human health by the infection or illness rates, based on given densities of particular pathogens, estimated or measured rates of ingestion and appropriate dose–response models for the exposed population. QMRA is usually done in four steps (Table 2.2). Examples of QMRAs used to estimate health risks associated with the use of excreta and greywater in agriculture are presented in chapter 3.

Hazard identification and problem formulation constitute the initial systematic planning step that identifies the goals and focus of the risk assessment and also may include the regulatory and policy context of the assessment.

Table 2.2 QMRA paradigm for quantifiable human health effects

Step	Aim
1. Hazard identification	To describe acute and chronic human health effects associated with any particular hazard, including pathogens or toxic chemicals
2. Hazard characterization	Dose–response assessment, to characterize the relationship between various doses administered and the incidence of the health effect, including underlying mechanisms and extrapolation from model systems to humans
3. Exposure assessment	To determine the size and nature of the population exposed and the route, amount and duration of the exposure
4. Risk characterization	To integrate the information from exposure assessment, hazard characterization and hazard identification steps in order to estimate the magnitude of the public health problem and to evaluate variability and uncertainty

Source: Adapted from WHO (2003a).

In *hazard characterization*, exposure and health effects are described with background information on, for example, the pathogens relevant in a special surrounding or environment. It also includes the range of human diseases associated with the identified microorganisms (Haas, Rose & Gerba, 1999). A conceptual model is developed that describes the interactions of pathogens with the defined population as well as assumptions made and attempts to address specific questions and identify information needs.

The dose–response relationship between microbial agents and the infection rate in a population is seldom directly estimated but is usually based on human volunteer studies presented in the literature. A mathematical relationship is obtained between the dose and the probability of infection (Teunis et al., 1996; Haas, Rose & Gerba, 1999), where either exponential (#1 in Box 2.2) or β-Poisson (#2 in Box 2.2) relationships are applied.

Exposure assessment describes the size and nature of the exposed population, as well as the duration or frequency of exposure and the exposure pathways. Elements involved are:

- pathogen characterization: determining the properties of the pathogen that affects its ability to be transmitted to and cause disease in the host;
- pathogen occurrence: characterizing the occurrence and distribution of the pathogen, including information on its ability to survive, persist and multiply.

The exposure profile provides a qualitative and/or quantitative description of the magnitude, frequency and patterns of exposure and a characterization of the source and temporal nature of the exposure. The dose of a pathogen is calculated from the density of the organism through the contact route multiplied by the volume ingested. Densities are either based on prevalence data for actual pathogens or indirectly estimated through index organisms (Ashbolt et al., 2006).

The analysis may also consider vulnerability and if and how social and/or behavioural traits influence susceptibility or severity. The clinical illness associated with the pathogen is summarized, including duration of clinical illness, mortality and sequelae.

The *risk characterization* integrates the information from the hazard identification, hazard characterization and exposure assessment to estimate the

Box 2.2 Example of mathematical determination of the dose–response relationship

Calculations are made as follows:

1) Random distribution and probability of infection for an organism equals r: $P_{inf} = 1 - e^{-rDose}$
2) Probability r not constant and has a distribution in itself (β-distribution) due to either the organism or the exposed population, where α and β describe the relation: $P_{inf} \approx 1 - (1 + Dose/\beta)^{-\alpha}$

The β-Poisson model fits well with many dose–response data sets and is conservative when extrapolating to low doses (Teunis et al., 1996), whereas the exponential relationship is applicable when dealing with pathogens where no dose response studies have been made, where vulnerable populations are exposed or in worst case scenarios (Figure 2.2). Then r = 1 can be applied as a generic single hit model, where ingestion, inhalation or contact with one organism will lead to $P_{inf} = 0.63$.

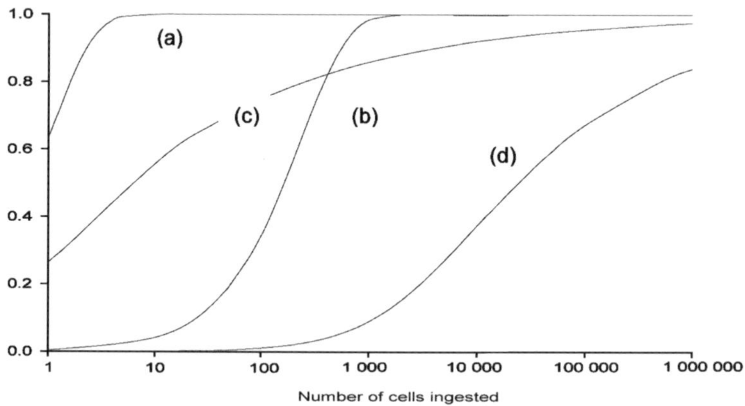

Figure 2.2
The probability of infection from the ingestion of pathogenic cells in different dose–response relationships: Exponential models for a) a worst-case scenario and b) *Cryptosporidium*; β-Poisson models for c) rotavirus and d) *Salmonella*

magnitude of the public health problem and to evaluate variability and uncertainty. Since information is usually incomplete and the density of pathogens fluctuates, probability density functions with Monte-Carlo simulations are better than point estimates or constant values in risk calculations. The microbial risk (probability of infection, P_{inf}) is presented either as the rate of infected people out of the number of exposed people or as the total number of infections per annum or system lifetime (Fane, Ashbolt & White, 2002). From a management point of view, the performance and reliability of a system might be more important than the absolute number of infections.

2.5 Tolerable risk and health-based targets

An important distinction needs to be made between the tolerable risk level of infection and the risk of disease. A number of factors determine whether infection with a specific pathogen will lead to a disease (virulence, the immune status of an individual, etc.). For example, hepatitis A infections in children are predominantly asymptomatic, but the same infection in adults often leads to clinical symptoms. Since rate of infection is harder to detect than disease symptoms, the relationship to health targets is more easily based on disease.

2.5.1 Tolerable risk

Risk assessments relate to health targets. A tolerable risk level is determined by a competent national authority or decided politically. The definition of what is tolerable may be based on the current prevalence of faecal–oral disease in a given population and to what extent this level will significantly decrease or increase due to the use of excreta and greywater in agriculture. Tolerable risk can be looked at in the context of total risk from all exposures, and risk management decisions can be used to address the greatest risks first. Tolerable risks can be set with the idea of continuous adaptation and improvement.

For carcinogenic chemicals in drinking-water, guideline values have been set at a 10^{-5} upper-bound estimate of risk (WHO, 2004a). This means that there would be a maximum of one excess case of cancer per 100 000 of the population ingesting drinking-water that contained the chemical at the guideline concentration over a lifetime. The disease burden associated with this level of risk and adjusted for the severity of the illness is approximately 1×10^{-6} DALY (1 µDALY) (WHO, 2004a). This level of disease burden can be compared with a mild but more frequent illness, such as self-limiting diarrhoea caused by a microbial pathogen. The estimated disease burden associated with mild diarrhoea (e.g. with a case fatality rate of $\sim 1 \times 10^{-5}$) at an annual disease risk of 1 in 1000 (10^{-3}) (~1 in 10 lifetime risk) is also about 1×10^{-6} DALY (1 µDALY) (WHO, 2004a).

2.5.2 Health-based targets

Health-based targets should be part of overall public health policy, taking into account status and trends and the contribution of the use of treated excreta or greywater in agriculture to the transmission of infectious disease both in individual settings and within overall health management. The purpose of setting targets is to mark out milestones to guide and chart progress towards a predetermined health goal. To ensure effective health protection and improvement, targets need to be realistic and relevant to local conditions and may also relate directly to the management strategies. This normally implies periodic review and updating of priorities and targets and, in turn, that norms and standards should be revised to take account of these factors and the changes in available information (WHO, 2004a).

A health-based target uses the tolerable risk of disease as a baseline to set specific performance targets that will reduce the risk of disease to this level. Exposure through different transmission routes to different concentrations of pathogens is associated with a certain level of risk. Reducing this risk thus involves reducing the levels of exposure or concentration of pathogens.

Health-based targets can be specified in terms of combinations of different components or single parameters, including:

- *Health outcome*: as determined by epidemiological studies, public health surveillance or QMRA (DALYs or absence of a specific disease);
- *Excreta or greywater quality*: e.g. concentrations of viable intestinal nematode eggs and/or *E. coli*;
- *Performance*: e.g. a performance target for removal of pathogens through a combination of treatment requirements, handling practices and quality

standards (chapters 4 and 5). Performance may be approximated by other parameters: storage time, temperature, etc.;
- *Specified technology*: specified treatment processes, either in general or with reference to specific circumstances of use.

2.6 Risk management

Health targets relate to certain basic control approaches. Risk management requires an assessment of the health risks at key points of the excreta or greywater use process (generation, point of use, final product consumption). Risk management strategies address controllable factors, such as:

- behaviours (e.g. hand washing with soap; adding lime to faeces);
- treatment technologies;
- operational processes: application to fields; operation and maintenance of facilities;
- protective action: cooking food properly prior to consumption; wearing protective clothing when coming into contact with wastes.

To best protect public health, multiple strategies may be needed simultaneously to add additional barriers to the transmission of disease.

The impacts of risk management actions can be measured only if the baseline health status of the affected population is known or can be approximated. Similarly, tolerable risk and health-based targets can be set only with some knowledge of the incidence and prevalence of infection and disease in the community, the types of diseases that may result from the use of excreta and greywater and the vulnerability of different subsections of the population (e.g. people with reduced immune function or those susceptible to specific hazards).

Initial information on background levels of faecal–oral disease in the population might be based on information collected from local health-care facilities, public health surveillance, laboratory analysis, epidemiological studies or specific research conducted in a project area. Infectious disease outbreaks provide additional information. There may be seasonal fluctuations in disease incidence — for example, during the wet season or cold season (e.g. rotavirus infections peak in the cold season) — which should be considered. In evaluating the use of excreta and greywater in a certain area, knowledge of disease trends (i.e. whether disease incidence is decreasing or increasing) is valuable. High background disease levels (e.g. intestinal worm infections) or disease outbreaks (e.g. cholera) might indicate that risk management procedures were not being implemented adequately and would need to be strengthened or reconsidered.

Risk management strategies for excreta and greywater aim at minimizing exposures to pathogens by multiple barriers. They may include combinations of the following:

- on-site storage and treatment to reduce pathogens to a level that presents a tolerable risk;
- off-site additional treatment for further pathogen reduction;
- crop restriction: growing crops that either are not eaten or are processed (cooked) prior to consumption;
- application techniques of excreta and greywater that reduce exposure of workers and contamination of crops (including withholding periods, buffer zones);

- exposure control methods: limiting public access; workers wearing protective clothing; washing, disinfecting and/or cooking food properly prior to consumption.

Information concerning the efficiency of processes in preventing exposures combined with data on the occurrence of pathogens enables the definition of operating conditions that would reasonably be expected to achieve those targets. Overall, the relatively greatest emphasis should be given to periodic inspection/auditing and to simple measurements that can be deployed rapidly and frequently and will directly inform management.

2.7 Public health status

In many countries, excreta and wastewater contain high concentrations of pathogens, and excreta-related infections are common. The failure to properly treat and manage wastewater and excreta worldwide is directly responsible for adverse health and environmental effects. Human excreta have been implicated in the transmission of many infectious diseases, including cholera, typhoid, types of viral hepatitis, polio, schistosomiasis and a variety of helminth infections. Most of these excreta-related illnesses occur in children living in poor countries. Overall, WHO estimates that diarrhoea alone is responsible for 3.2% of all deaths and 4.2% of DALYs worldwide (WHO, 2004b). In addition to diarrhoea, WHO estimates that each year, 16 million people contract typhoid and over 1 billion people suffer from intestinal helminth infections (WHO, 2000, 2003b, 2003c, 2004b). Diarrhoea or gastrointestinal disease is often used as a proxy for all excreta-related infectious diseases. Mead et al. (1999) estimated that the average person (including all age groups) in the USA suffers from 0.79 episode of acute gastroenteritis (characterized by diarrhoea, vomiting or both) per year. The rates of acute gastroenteritis among adults worldwide are generally within the same order of magnitude. However, children — especially those living in

Table 2.3 Global mortality and DALYs due to some diseases of relevance to excreta and wastewater use

Disease	Mortality (deaths/year)	Burden of disease (DALYs/year)	Comments
Diarrhoea	1 798 000	61 966 000	99.8% of deaths occur in developing countries; 90% of deaths occur in children
Typhoid	600 000	N/A	Estimated 16 million cases per year
Ascariasis	3 000	1 817 000	Estimated 1.45 billion infections, of which 350 million suffer adverse health effects
Hookworm disease	3 000	59 000	Estimated 1.3 billion infections, of which 150 million suffer adverse health effects
Schistosomiasis	15 000	1 702 000	Found in 74 countries, 200 million people worldwide are estimated to be infected, 20 million with severe consequences
Hepatitis A	N/A	N/A	Estimated 1.4 million cases per year worldwide; serological evidence of prior infection ranges from 15% to nearly 100%

N/A = not available
Sources: WHO (2000, 2003b, 2003c, 2004b).

high-risk situations, where poor hygiene, lack of access to sanitation and poor water quality prevail — generally have a higher rate of gastrointestinal illness. Kosek, Bern & Guerrant (2003) found that children under the age of five in developing countries experienced a median of 3.2 episodes of diarrhoea per child per year.

Table 2.3 provides estimates of mortality and morbidity for some diseases of possible relevance to excreta and greywater use in agriculture.

3
ASSESSMENT OF HEALTH RISK

The use of excreta and greywater in agriculture has the potential for both positive and negative health consequences. Positive health benefits may arise from the safe use of treated excreta and greywater, especially when these activities increase household food security, increase nutritional variety and/or generate household income that can be used to support health-promoting activities such as education or access to better health care. These benefits, however, have rarely been quantified in a systematic way. The value of using excreta as a fertilizer has been described in chapter 1.

The negative health consequences relate to the transmission of infectious diseases through improper management of excreta and greywater and, to a lesser extent, exposure to chemicals. This chapter presents an overview of organisms found in faeces and urine that are of public health importance. The microbial risks in relation to greywater relate to the load of faecal material, which is much lower than in wastewater. Easily degradable organic material may promote regrowth of indicator bacteria in greywater, which is briefly described. The risks to consumers are dealt with from an epidemiological perspective. The chapter also summarizes existing information on the survival/die-off of pathogens in faeces, urine and greywater systems, which forms an integrated concept in risk assessment. The assessment of health risk, following the procedure outlined in the Stockholm Framework (see chapter 2), is exemplified for faeces, urine and greywater.

3.1 Health benefits

The health benefits from excreta are linked mainly to their value as fertilizer to enhance crop productivity and thus the availability of agricultural products. Excreta use as fertilizer has so far been mainly applied in small-scale applications in rural areas and urban agriculture, as described in chapter 1. Greywater is used mainly for irrigation, similarly benefiting crop production. It is an important resource for the poor in water-scarce areas and elsewhere. Indirect health benefits also relate to its economic value (chapter 9) and reduced environmental impact (chapter 8). Although the benefits of excreta as a fertilizer are well established, the role of greywater is less well characterized in this respect.

Improving nutrition is critical for maintaining the overall health of individuals and communities, especially for children. Malnutrition is estimated to play a significant role in the deaths of 50% of all children in developing countries (10.4 million children under the age of five die per year) (Rice et al., 2000; WHO, 2000). Malnutrition affects approximately 800 million people (20% of all people) in the developing world (WHO, 2000). Excreta and greywater, as readily available sources of plant fertilizer, can help to alleviate malnutrition if managed well, yet they also can cause malnutrition (e.g. iron deficiency anaemia) through hookworm infection if proper risk management strategies are not employed (see chapter 5).

Combining poverty, malnutrition and lack of access to safe drinking-water and adequate sanitation into one picture shows a downward spiral, which, at the individual level, comes to expression in the following phenomena:

- Poor people may eat and absorb too little nutritious food and be more disease-prone.
- Inadequate or inappropriate food leads to stunted development (one in three children under the age of five in the developing world are stunted) and/or premature death.
- Nutrient-deficient diets provoke health problems (100–140 million children are vitamin A deficient; 4–5 billion people are affected by iron deficiency; and 2 billion people are anaemic); malnutrition increases susceptibility to disease.

- The immune system is unable to adequately cope with often multiple infections.
- Disease decreases people's ability to cultivate or purchase nutritious foods.

Therefore, resources (including excreta and greywater) that improve the household's ability to produce or purchase sufficient quantities of nutritious food can impact health at the individual and community levels.

3.2 Excreta-related infections

The first step of any risk assessment is hazard identification. For risk assessment of excreta-related infections, the pathogens relevant in a specific setting under specific conditions or associated with specific actions are identified. The associated infections are common in the human population in many countries with correspondingly high concentrations of excreted pathogens.

Several factors govern the likelihood of pathogen transmission:

- epidemiological features (including infectious dose, latency, hosts and intermediate host);
- persistence in different environments outside the human body (and potential for growth);
- major transmission routes;
- relative susceptibility to different treatment techniques;
- management control measures.

These factors are accounted for in the hazard identification step. The relevant microbial agents are identified, as well as the spectrum of human ill-health associated with each pathogen. Acquired immunity and multiple exposures (e.g. exposure at different times or through different routes) need to be considered. Since it is not feasible to assess the potential impact of all excreta-related pathogens, some are commonly chosen as indicator pathogens (when their reduction due to different barriers is assessed, the term "index pathogens" is often used).

The prevalence of excreta-related pathogens in a human population is a measure of their presence in the environment. Key factors to be considered at the stage of hazard identification are, therefore:

- disease prevalence and incidence (if possible, corrected for underreporting);
- percentage of infections leading to disease (morbidity, differs between organisms);
- excretion density (differs between organisms);
- excretion time and prevalence of asymptomatic carriers (differs between organisms);
- excretion route (faeces or urine).

The disease prevalence rate is the number of clinical cases caused by a specific pathogen at a specific moment in time, usually standardized to the number of cases per 100 000. The disease incidence rate is the number of new cases divided by the total population over a period of time, usually one year and usually standardized to the number of new cases per 100 000 people over that period. Incidence will vary in accordance with the prevailing epidemiological situation in a given area. The reported number of cases is, however, often substantially underestimated, since the infected person must be symptomatic, recognized in the medical care system with the right diagnosis and reported. Estimates of underreporting (i.e. how many more cases exist in the community than were reported) are presented in Table 3.1. Generally, pathogens causing less severe symptoms are less likely to be reported (Wheeler et al., 1999).

Table 3.1 Examples of different epidemiological data for selected pathogens

Pathogen	Incidence (per 100 000 people)	Under-reporting	Morbidity (%)	Excretion (per gram faeces)	Duration (days)	ID_{50}
Salmonella	42–58	3.2	6–80	10^{4-8}	26–51	23 600
Campylobacter	78–97	7.6	25	10^{6-9}	1–77	900
EHEC	0.8–1.4	4.5–8.3	76–89	10^{2-3}	5–12	1 120
Hepatitis A virus	0.8–7.8	3	70	10^{4-6}	13–30	30
Rotavirus	21	35	50	10^{7-11}	1–39	6
Norovirus	1.2	1562	70	10^{5-9}	5–22	10
Adenovirus	300	–	54	–	1–14	1.7
Cryptosporidium	0.3–1.6	4–19	39	10^{7-8}	2–30	165
Giardia	15–26	20	20–40	10^{5-8}	28–284	35
Ascaris	15–25	–	15	10^{4}	107–557	0.7

Source: Westrell (2004).

The infection prevalence and amount of faeces excreted will determine the pathogen concentration at the time of excretion. The subsequent risks will relate to (1) their persistence (or regrowth or environmental latency), which will vary in relation to the receiving environment and the organism in question, (2) dilution factors (e.g. the amount of human faeces that will end up in greywater), (3) exposure route (and frequency of exposure) and (4) dose (i.e. the amount of material, and thus the number of pathogens, to which a person is exposed). Risks will vary due to the infectious dose of the organism in question and the vulnerability of the exposed population. In order for a person to become infected when exposed to a pathogen, the pathogen must breach the host's defence mechanisms. The median infectious dose, ID_{50}, is the pathogen dose at which 50% of a population will be infected. An infected person excretes pathogens, often in very high numbers and for many days (Table 3.1). Not all infections are symptomatic, however. Morbidity is a measure of the percentage of people who will show clinical symptoms when infected.

Values in Table 3.1 are taken from developed regions. The incidence data for norovirus and adenovirus are based on Wheeler et al. (1999) and for *Ascaris* on Arnbjerg-Nielsen et al. (2004) in Denmark, with corresponding values for underreporting (Mead et al., 1999; Wheeler et al., 1999; Michel et al., 2000; Carrique-Mas et al., 2003) and morbidity (Feachem et al., 1983; Van et al, 1992; Graham et al., 1994; Gerba et al., 1996; Lemon, 1997; Haas, Rose & Gerba, 1999; Tessier & Davies, 1999; Havelaar, de Wit & van Koningsveld, 2000; Michel et al., 2000).

3.2.1 Pathogens in faeces

Enteric infections can be transmitted by pathogenic species of bacteria, viruses, parasitic protozoa and helminths. From a risk perspective, exposure to untreated faeces is always considered unsafe, due to the potential presence of high levels of pathogens, depending on their prevalence in a given population.

Enteric bacterial pathogens continue to be of major concern, especially in developing countries, where outbreaks of cholera, typhoid and shigellosis appear to be more frequent in urban and periurban areas. In areas where access to adequate sanitation is non-existent or insufficient, typhoid fever (*Salmonella typhi*) and cholera (*Vibrio cholerae*) constitute major risks through the resulting contamination of drinking-water. *Shigella* is a common cause of diarrhoea in developing countries, especially in settings where hygiene and sanitation are poor. Among the bacteria, at least *Salmonella*, *Campylobacter* and enterohaemorrhagic *E. coli* (EHEC) are of general importance, both in industrialized and in developing countries, from the perspective of microbial risks posed by the use of various fertilizer products (including faeces, sewage sludge and animal manure). These bacteria are also important as zoonotic agents (transmission between humans and animals, with contamination from faeces/manure).

Enteric viruses are also of general importance and are now considered to be the cause of the majority of gastrointestinal infections in industrialized regions (Svensson, 2000). Of the different types of viruses that may be excreted in faeces, the most common are members included in the enterovirus, rotavirus, enteric adenovirus and human calicivirus (norovirus) groups (Tauxe & Cohen, 1995). Hepatitis A virus has long been recognized as being of major concern when applying wastes to land and is considered a risk for both water- and foodborne outbreaks, especially when the sanitary standards are low. Recognition of the importance of hepatitis E virus is emerging.

The parasitic protozoa *Cryptosporidium parvum* and *Giardia intestinalis* have been studied intensively during the last decade, partly due to their high environmental persistence and low infectious doses. *Cryptosporidium* is associated with several large waterborne outbreaks, and *Giardia* is occurring with high prevalence as an enteric pathogen. *Entamoeba histolytica* is also recognized as an infectious agent of concern in developing countries. The global importance of other protozoa, such as *Cyclospora* and *Isospora*, is currently being debated.

In developing countries, geohelminth infections are of major concern. The eggs (ova) of, especially, *Ascaris* and *Taenia* are persistent in the environment and are therefore regarded as an indicator and index of hygienic quality (WHO, 1989). Hookworm disease is widespread in most tropical and subtropical areas and affects nearly one billion people worldwide. In some developing countries, these infections exacerbate malnutrition and indirectly cause the death of many children by increasing their susceptibility to other infections.

Of the parasitic trematode worms causing schistosomiasis, the eggs of one species, *Schistosoma haematobium*, are excreted predominantly in urine (see below), whereas the eggs of the other species (*S. japonicum*, *S. mansoni* and *S. mekongi*) are excreted in faeces. They also differ in their geographical distribution. *S. japonicum* occurs in the Western Pacific Region (mainly China and the Philippines), *S. mekongi* in foci in the Mekong River basin, *S. haematobium* in Africa and the Eastern Mediterranean Region and *S. mansoni* in Africa and in parts of Central and South America, notably Brazil (WHO, 2003a). More than 200 million people are currently infected with schistosomiasis. The use of treated excreta should not pose a risk, but the use of fresh or untreated faecal material does, if it happens close to freshwater sources where the intermediate host snail species are present.

The pathogens whose transmission can be attributed to the use of faecal excreta mainly cause gastrointestinal symptoms such as diarrhoea, vomiting and stomach

Table 3.2 Examples of pathogens that may be excreted in faeces and related diseases and symptoms

Group	Pathogen	Disease and symptoms
Bacteria	*Aeromonas* spp.	Enteritis
	Campylobacter jejuni/coli	Campylobacteriosis – diarrhoea, cramps, abdominal pains, fever, nausea, arthritis; Guillain-Barré syndrome
	Escherichia coli (EIEC, EPEC, ETEC, EHEC)	Enteritis
	Plesiomonas shigelloides	Enteritis
	Salmonella typhi/paratyphi	Typhoid/paratyphoid fever – headache, fever, malaise, anorexia, bradycardia, splenomegaly, cough
	Salmonella spp.	Salmonellosis – diarrhoea, fever, abdominal cramps
	Shigella spp.	Shigellosis – dysentery (bloody diarrhoea), vomiting, cramps, fever; Reiter's syndrome
	Vibrio cholerae	Cholera – watery diarrhoea, lethal if severe and untreated
	Yersinia spp.	Yersiniosis – fever, abdominal pain, diarrhoea, joint pains, rash
Viruses	Enteric adenovirus 40 and 41	Enteritis
	Astrovirus	Enteritis
	Calicivirus (including norovirus)	Enteritis
	Coxsackievirus	Various: respiratory illness; enteritis; viral meningitis
	Echovirus	Aseptic meningitis; encephalitis; often asymptomatic
	Enterovirus types 68–71	Meningitis; encephalitis; paralysis
	Hepatitis A virus	Hepatitis – fever, malaise, anorexia, nausea, abdominal discomfort, jaundice
	Hepatitis E virus	Hepatitis
	Poliovirus	Poliomyelitis – often asymptomatic, fever, nausea, vomiting, headache, paralysis
	Rotavirus	Enteritis
Parasitic protozoa	*Cryptosporidium parvum*	Cryptosporidiosis – watery diarrhoea, abdominal cramps and pain
	Cyclospora cayetanensis	Often asymptomatic; diarrhoea, abdominal pain
	Entamoeba histolytica	Amoebiasis – often asymptomatic; dysentery, abdominal discomfort, fever, chills
	Giardia intestinalis	Giardiasis – diarrhoea, abdominal cramps, malaise, weight loss
Helminths	*Ascaris lumbricoides* (roundworm)	Ascariasis – generally no or few symptoms; wheezing, coughing, fever, enteritis, pulmonary eosinophilia
	Taenia solium/saginata (tapeworm)	Taeniasis
	Trichuris trichiura (whipworm)	Trichuriasis – Unapparent through vague digestive tract distress to emaciation with dry skin and diarrhoea
	Ancylostoma duodenale / Necator americanus (hookworm)	Itch, rash, cough, anaemia, protein deficiency
	Schistosoma spp. (blood fluke)	Schistosomiasis, bilharzia

Source: Adapted from Ottosson (2003).

cramps. Several may also cause symptoms involving other organs and severe sequelae. Table 3.2 lists the main pathogens of concern and the symptoms they cause.

3.2.2 Pathogens in urine

Environmental transmission of urinary excreted pathogens is of limited concern in temperate climates, but any faecal cross-contamination that may occur will end up diluted in the urine and may subsequently pose a health risk. In tropical climates, faecal contamination of collected urine is considered the main risk, but some urine-excreted pathogens also need to be considered. The risk of pathogen transmission during handling, transportation and reuse of diverted urine is, however, mainly based on the amount of faecal material contaminating the urine fraction.

Traditional faecal indicators such as *E. coli* are not useful for monitoring faecal contamination of urine due to their short survival time in urine. Faecal streptococci may be used as a "storage indicator" but are able to regrow in the pipes of larger urine diversion systems. Studies conducted with chemical indicators of faecal contamination (faecal sterols) indicate that faecal amounts are normally low, but contamination does occur in a significant proportion of urine diversion schemes. For example, 22–37% of urine or sludge from urine storage tanks indicated slight faecal contamination (Schönning, Leeming & Stenström, 2002). Samples collected from systems where there were several user families (small communities or apartment blocks) were more frequently contaminated than samples from individual households.

In a healthy individual, urine in the bladder is sterile. However, different types of bacteria are picked up in the urinary tract. Freshly excreted urine normally contains <10 000 bacteria per ml. In urinary tract infections, significantly higher amounts of bacteria are excreted. These are normally not transmitted to other individuals through the environment. Sexually transmitted pathogens may occasionally be excreted in urine, but there is no evidence that their potential survival outside the body would be of public health importance.

Some pathogens, such as *Leptospira interrogans*, *Salmonella typhi*, *Salmonella paratyphi*, *Schistosoma haematobium* and some viruses, are excreted in urine. A range of other pathogens have been detected in urine, but further risk of environmental transmission may be considered insignificant.

Leptospirosis is a bacterial infection causing influenza-like symptoms and is in general transmitted by urine from infected animals (Feachem et al., 1983; CDC, 2003). It is considered an occupational hazard, for example, for sewage workers and for farm workers in developing countries (CDC, 2003). In tropical and subtropical climates, this disease is important in domestic animals, both for the risk to humans and due to economic losses. It is a severe disease with a 5–10% mortality rate (Olsson Engvall & Gustavsson, 2001). The bacteria survive for several months in freshwater and moist environments at neutral pH and at temperatures around 25 °C. Leptospiral bacteria in urine-contaminated environments enter a host through the mucous membranes and through small abrasions in the skin. Human urine is not considered to provide an important transmission pathway for leptospirosis due to low prevalence (Feachem et al., 1983; CDC, 2003).

Persons infected with *S. typhi* and *S. paratyphi* excrete the organisms in urine during the phase of typhoid and paratyphoid fevers when bacteria are disseminated in the blood. Even though the infection is endemic in several developing countries, with an estimated 16 million cases per year, urine–oral transmission is probably unusual compared with faecal–oral transmission. For diverted urine, the risk for further transmission of *Salmonella* is low, even with short storage times, due to the rapid inactivation of Gram-negative faecal bacteria (Höglund, 2001). Die-off rates of *Salmonella* spp. are rapid and similar to those for *E. coli* in collected urine.

Persons infected with *Schistosoma haematobium* excrete the eggs in urine, sometimes for extended periods of time. The eggs hatch in the freshwater environment, and the larvae (miracidia) infect the intermediate hosts, specific aquatic snails of the genus *Bulinus*. The parasites transform and multiply inside the snail, which then sheds the next stage of aquatic larvae (cercariae). These may infect humans in contact with water by penetrating the skin. If the eggs do not reach freshwater bodies where the snail intermediate host is present within days, the infectious cycle is broken, which is the case if the urine is stored for days and is used on arable land. Fresh urine should not be used close to surface waters in endemic areas.

Mycobacterium tuberculosis and *Mycobacterium bovis* may be excreted in urine (Bentz et al., 1975; Grange & Yates, 1992). *M. tuberculosis* has occasionally been isolated in excreta and greywater from hospitals (Dailloux et al., 1999). Humans are able to infect cattle with both the bovine and the human strain, and individuals on farms have transmitted bovine tuberculosis to cattle by urinating in cowsheds (Huitema, 1969; Collins & Grange, 1987). It is, however, unlikely that transmission of either human or bovine tuberculosis is significantly affected by exposure to urine (or faeces). Other mycobacterial species (atypical mycobacteria) may also be isolated from urine. They are widely distributed in the environment and commonly found in waters, including as contaminants in drinking-water (Grange & Yates, 1992; Dailloux et al., 1999).

Microsporidia are a group of protozoa implicated in human disease, mainly in HIV-positive individuals (Marshall et al., 1997; Cotte et al., 1999). The infective spores are shed in faeces and urine, with consequences for possible environmental transmission (Haas, Rose & Gerba, 1999). Microsporidia have been found in sewage and water. Water- or foodborne outbreaks have been suspected but are not well documented (Cotte et al., 1999; Haas, Rose & Gerba, 1999).

Cytomegalovirus is excreted in urine, but it is a person-to-person transmitted disease and not considered to be spread by food and water (Jawetz, Melnick & Adelberg, 1987). Two polyomaviruses, JC virus (JCV) and BK virus (BKV), are also excreted in urine (Bofill-Mas, Pina & Girones, 2000). Both have been found in sewage in various countries. Even if the viruses occur in excreta, transmission to humans by this route is unlikely. Infections will occur mainly through close contacts within or outside the family at a young age (Kunitake et al., 1995; Bofill-Mas, Pina & Girones, 2000). In one Japanese investigation, it was found that 46% of persons aged 20–29 years excreted urinary JCV (Kitamura et al., 1994).

One foodborne outbreak of hepatitis A caused by lettuce contaminated by urine has been reported (Ollinger-Snyder & Matthews, 1996). Hepatitis B virus has also been found in human urine, with potential further transmission in hyperendemic areas (Knutsson & Kidd-Ljunggren, 2000). Adenovirus may also be excreted in urine, especially from children with haemorrhagic cystitis, transplant patients and HIV-positive individuals (Mufson & Belshe, 1976; Shields et al., 1985; Echavarria et al., 1998). However, the public health significance from urinary transmission has not been established.

It can be concluded that pathogens that may be transmitted through urine (Table 3.3) are rarely sufficiently common to constitute a significant public health problem and are not considered to constitute a health risk in the reuse of human urine in temperate climates. *Schistosoma haematobium* is an exception in tropical areas, however, with a low risk of transmission due to its life cycle.

Table 3.3 Pathogens that may be excreted in urine and the importance of urine as a transmission route

Pathogen	Urine as a transmission route	Importance
Leptospira interrogans	Usually through animal urine	Probably low
Salmonella typhi and *Salmonella paratyphi*	Probably unusual, excreted in urine in systemic infection	Low compared with other transmission routes
Schistosoma haematobium (eggs excreted)	Not directly but indirectly, larvae infect humans in fresh water	Needs to be considered in endemic areas where snail intermediate hosts are present
Mycobacteria	Unusual, usually airborne	Low
Viruses: cytomegalovirus, polyomaviruses JCV, BKV, adenovirus, hepatitis virus and others	Not normally recognized other than single cases of hepatitis A and suggested for hepatitis B; more information needed	Probably low
Microsporidia	Incriminated, but not confirmed	Low
Sexually transmitted pathogens	No, do not survive for significant periods outside the body	Insignificant
Urinary tract infections	No, no direct environmental transmission	Low to insignificant

The main risks in the use of excreta are related to the faecal and not the urinary fraction. Reducing faecal cross-contamination of the urine fraction is therefore an important control measure. Even though some pathogens may be excreted in urine, the faecal cross-contamination that may occur by misplacement of faeces in a urine-diverting toilet is associated with the most significant health risks (Höglund, Ashbolt & Stenström, 2002).

3.2.3 Pathogens in greywater

Interest in reusing greywater has increased in recent years, especially in arid areas. In some densely populated areas, such as Singapore and Tokyo, greywater reuse including different system approaches and treatment alternatives is a common practice (Asano & Levine, 1996; Jeppesen, 1996; Trujillo et al., 1998; Dixon, Butler & Fewkes, 1999; Shrestha, Haberl & Laber, 2001). In source separating systems, opportunistic pathogenic bacteria may emanate from growth within the actual system or from washing, kitchen activities or personal hygiene.

In buildings, opportunistic pathogenic bacteria, such as *Legionella*, mycobacteria and *Pseudomonas aeruginosa*, may grow. The risk is probably not greater than from exposure to hot tap water.

The main hazards of greywater originate from faecal cross-contamination (section 3.2.2). Faecal contamination is limited and related to activities such as washing faecally contaminated laundry (i.e. diapers), child care, anal cleansing and showering. Faecal contamination is measured traditionally by the use of common indicator organisms, such as coliforms and enterococci. This method has also been applied for assessing faecal contamination of greywater (Table 3.4).

Table 3.4 Reported numbers of indicator bacteria in greywater

Excreta and greywater origin	Numbers of indicator bacteria (log numbers/100 ml)				Reference
	Total coliforms	Thermotolerant coliforms	*E. coli*	Enterococci	
Bath, hand basin			4.4	1.0–5.4	Albrechtsen (1998)
Laundry	3.4–5.5	2.0–3.0		1.4–3.4	Christova-Boal, Eden & McFarlane (1996)
Shower, hand basin	2.7–7.4	2.2–3.5		1.9–3.4	Christova-Boal, Eden & McFarlane (1996)
Greywater	7.9	5.8		2.4	Casanova, Gerba & Karpiscak (2001)
Shower, bath	1.8–3.9	0–3.7		0–4.8	Feachem et al. (1983)
Laundry, wash	1.9–5.9	1.0–4.2		1.5–3.9	Feachem et al. (1983)
Laundry, rinse	2.3–5.2	0–5.4		0–6.1	Feachem et al. (1983)
Greywater	7.2–8.8				Gerba et al. (1995)
Hand basin, kitchen sink		5.0		4.6	Gunther (2000)
Greywater, 79% shower	7.4	4.3–6.9			Rose et al. (1991)
Kitchen sink		7.6	7.4	7.7	Naturvårdsverket (1995)
Greywater		5.8	5.4	4.6	Naturvårdsverket (1995)

Source: Ottosson (2003).

However, greywater may contain a high load of easily degradable organic compounds, which favours the growth of faecal indicators, as reported by Manville et al. (2001), in greywater systems. Hence, bacterial indicator numbers may lead to an overestimation of faecal loads and the associated risk. Occasionally, enteric pathogenic bacteria, such as *Salmonella* and *Campylobacter*, can be introduced by inadequate food handling in the kitchen (Cogan, Bloomfield & Humphrey, 1999), in addition to faecal matter derived directly from humans. The individual risk is higher from the direct handling of the contaminated food, but limited to a few exposed persons in the individual household, whereas a larger number of people may be exposed with reused greywater as the source. There is also a risk of regrowth of some pathogenic bacteria within the greywater system itself.

3.3 Pathogen survival in faeces, urine and greywater

3.3.1 Survival in faeces

Feachem et al. (1983) compiled extensive literature data on pathogen/indicator reductions in different materials, including nightsoil and faeces. The data were presented as "less than" values and did not consider the initial concentrations and die-off rate, but rather total inactivation. An additional compilation (Schönning et al., 2006) estimated the decimal reduction times for selected pathogens, but recent data on pathogen inactivation in human faeces are limited. If the initial concentrations are high and first-order die-off kinetics are applied, the time for total die-off is longer than in Feachem et al. (1983). However, this is not necessarily applicable during extended storage. Additional information was drawn from similar investigations of the die-off of selected pathogens in animal manure, animal slurry and sewage sludge (Arnbjerg-Nielsen et al., 2004), with its corresponding values after incorporation into soil (Table 3.5) and expressed as time for 90% inactivation (T_{90} values).

Table 3.5 Die-off of selected pathogens in faeces and soil, expressed as T_{90} values

	T_{90} faeces (days, mean ± standard deviation)	T_{90} soil (days, mean ± standard deviation)
Salmonella	30 ± 8	35 ± 6
EHEC	20 ± 4	25 ± 6
Rotavirus	60 ± 16	30 ± 8
Hepatitis A virus	55 ± 18	75 ± 10
Giardia	27.5 ± 9	30 ± 4
Cryptosporidium	70 ± 20	495 ± 182
Ascaris	125 ± 30	625 ± 150

The number of pathogens in faecal material will be reduced with time during storage due to natural die-off, without further treatment. The type of organism and storage conditions govern the time-dependent reduction or elimination. Ambient temperature, pH, moisture and biological competition will all affect inactivation. Variations in storage conditions will reflect in the die-off rates.

In a South African study, *Salmonella* was found in stored faeces after one year (Austin, 2001). Wood ash sprinkled over the faeces gave a pH of 8.6–9.4. The material had been partially wetted, and *Salmonella* could have grown in the material. Weekly turnings of the faecal heap resulted in a high reduction in pathogen numbers and faecal indicators and low moisture (Austin, 2001). Aeration increases inactivation, since a partial composting may have taken place (temperature not reported).

In a Danish study, the risks related to the use of faeces that had been stored for up to 12 months without additional treatment were calculated (Schönning et al., in press). *Ascaris* posed the highest risk, with a high likelihood of infecting vulnerable persons after accidental ingestion of the material. The protozoa (*Giardia* and *Cryptosporidium*) and rotavirus also resulted in high risks after accidental ingestion during handling or using unstored faeces in the gardens. After storage for 6 months, the risk was extrapolated to be 10%, whereas after 12 months, it was typically around 1:1000. The risk for hepatitis A or bacterial infections was generally lower. The storage was assumed to occur at about 10 °C.

In a study in Mexico (Franzén & Skott, 1999) with faecal material (moisture 10%, pH around 8, temperature 20–24 °C), a conservative viral indicator was added in controlled amounts and was reduced 1.5 log units after six weeks of storage. Low moisture content had a beneficiary reduction effect on added bacteriophages in latrines in Viet Nam (Carlander & Westrell, 1999). These latrines also had a pH of around 9, but higher temperatures (30–40 °C). A total inactivation of *Ascaris* was recorded within six months. This inactivation was not statistically related to any single factor in the latrines, but a combination of high temperature and high pH was suggested to account for the main reduction. Strauss & Blumenthal (1990) suggested that one year was sufficient for inactivation under tropical conditions (28–30 °C), whereas 18 months would be needed at lower temperatures (17–20 °C). This has also been supported by additional studies in Viet Nam (Phi et al., 2004).

In El Salvador, an extensive study of faecal material collected in urine-diverting toilets has been conducted. Material to increase the pH is added to the faecal material by the users, but the recording of some pH values around 6 implies that, in some toilets, only treatment by storage occurs (Moe & Izurieta, 2004). Survival analysis suggested that faecal coliforms would survive more than 1000 days and *Ascaris* around 600 days in latrines with a pH of less than 9!

Storage is especially beneficial in dry, hot climates, with desiccation of the material and low moisture contents aiding pathogen inactivation. If the faecal material is completely dry, the decrease in pathogen numbers is facilitated. Esrey et al. (1998) suggested that there is rapid pathogen destruction at moisture levels below 25% and that this level should be aimed for in ecological sanitation toilets that are based on dehydration (i.e. storage). Low moisture content is also beneficial in order to reduce odour and fly breeding (Esrey et al., 1998; Carlander & Westrell, 1999). Regrowth of bacterial pathogens may, however, occur after application of moisture or if the material is mixed with a moist soil. Desiccation is not a composting process; when moisture is added, the easily metabolized organic compounds will facilitate bacterial growth, including, for example, *E. coli* and *Salmonella*, if small amounts of these are occurring in or introduced into the material. Protozoan cysts are sensitive to desiccation, also affecting their survival on plant surfaces (Snowdon, Cliver & Converse, 1989; Yates & Gerba, 1998). Normal moisture levels do not inactivate *Ascaris* eggs. Moisture levels below 5% are needed to inactivate *Ascaris* eggs (Feachem et al., 1983), but the time required for inactivation is not known.

3.3.2 Survival in urine

For the hygienic risks related to the handling and reuse of urine, temperature, dilution, pH, ammonia and time are the main determinants affecting the persistence of organisms in collected urine. The technical design of the urine-diverting system (e.g. flushing and storage procedures) may also influence pathogen persistence.

The short survival of *E. coli* in urine makes it unsuitable as a general indicator for faecal contamination by, for example, viruses and protozoa. It is, however, representative for the die-off of Gram-negative bacteria. The T_{90} values were generally from <1 to 5 days, depending on the prevailing conditions; the longer times represent a pH value of 6. Longer persistence was also recorded if the urine was diluted 10-fold. Gram-negative bacteria such as *Campylobacter*, *Salmonella*, *Aeromonas hydrophila* and *Pseudomonas aeruginosa* were inactivated as rapidly as *E. coli*, indicating a low risk for transmission of bacterial gastrointestinal infections when handling diverted urine. The Gram-positive faecal streptococci had a longer survival (normally a T_{90} value of 4–7 days at 20 °C, but up to 30 days at 4 °C), and spore-forming clostridia were not reduced at all during a period of 80 days. In general, lower temperature and higher dilution result in longer survival of most bacteria. Extreme pH values were most deleterious. The rapid reduction of bacteria at high pH values is probably an effect both of the pH and of ammonia.

No significant inactivation of either rotavirus or a sentinel phage occurred at 5 °C during six months of storage, while the mean T_{90} values at 20 °C were estimated at 35 and 71 days for rotavirus and the phage, respectively (Figure 3.1). Rotavirus inactivation appeared to be largely temperature dependent, whereas there was an additional viricidal effect on the phage in urine at 20 °C (pH 9).

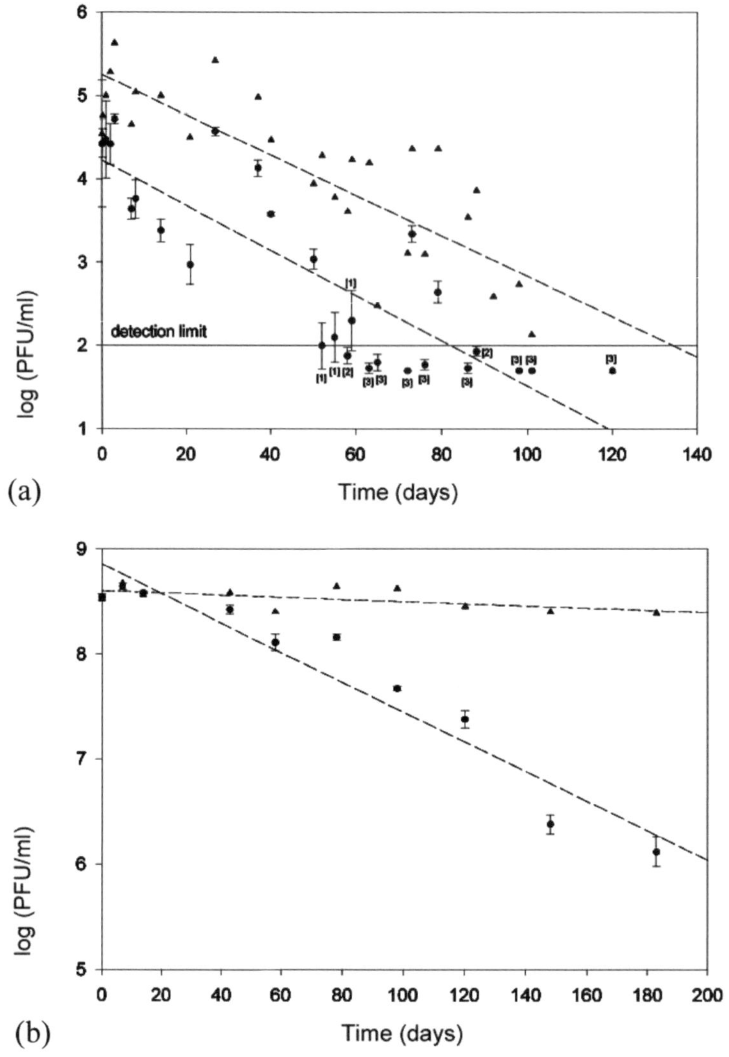

Figure 3.1
Inactivation of (a) rotavirus and (b) *Salmonella typhimurium* phage 28B in diverted human urine (•) and control medium (▲) at 20 °C (PFU = plaque-forming units)

Cryptosporidium parvum is known to be persistent in waste products as well as in water and to be resistant to disinfectants (Meinhardt, Casemore & Miller, 1996) and is a conservative index of protozoa in urine (Höglund & Stenström, 1999). In a urine mixture at pH 9 and 4 °C, the oocysts were inactivated to below the detection limit within about two months. The T_{90} value for *Cryptosporidium* was about one month at 4 °C and five days at 20 °C. The inactivation at pH 9 was significantly higher ($P < 0.01$) than at pH 5 and pH 7. The anti-protozoan effect of urine at pH 9 seems to be mediated by other factors besides the actual pH. Ammonia (NH_3) has been demonstrated to act as an inactivating agent for *Cryptosporidium* (Jenkins, Bowman & Ghiorse, 1998). The concentration of free ammonia (NH_3) in urine (pH 9, 4 °C) was about 0.03 mol/l (Höglund & Stenström, 1999).

In summary, Gram-negative bacteria are rapidly inactivated, while oocysts of *Cryptosporidium parvum* are reduced by approximately 90% per month in the urine mixture. Viruses are the most persistent group of microorganisms, with no inactivation in urine at 5 °C and T_{90} values of 35–71 days at 20 °C. Temperature may be considered the most important parameter (results summarized in Table 3.6). For bacteria, further dilution of the urine prolonged their survival. The effects of pH and ammonia are combined. However, rotavirus was not affected by pH or by ammonia. The information on helminths, including *Ascaris*, is limited and partly contradictory. According to Hamdy (1970), urine is ovicidal and *Ascaris* eggs are killed within hours; preliminary results from ongoing studies indicate that the reduction of *Ascaris suum* in urine is minor, with a 15–20% reduction during a 21-day period. Early studies also reported inactivation of *Schistosoma haematobium* in urine (Porter, 1938).

Table 3.6 Summarized results from survival experiments

	T_{90} values (days required for a 90% reduction)				
	Gram-negative bacteria	**Gram-positive bacteria**	***C. parvum***	**Rotavirus**	***S. typhimurium* phage 28B**
4 °C	1	30	29	172[a]	1466[a]
20 °C	1	5	5	35	71

[a] Survival experiments performed at 5 °C.

3.3.3 Faecal load and survival of faecal pathogens in greywater

The pathogen-related risks of greywater depend on the faecal load or faecal misplacement. The presence of degradable organic matter in greywater will support bacterial growth. Therefore, their numbers may lead to an overestimation of the risks. A number of faecal indicator organisms and biomarkers have been compared for a quantification of the faecal load in greywater (Ottosson, 2003) (Table 3.7), calculated as follows:

$$\frac{(\text{Microorganism density [numbers/ml]} \times \text{Flow [ml/person per day]})}{\text{Excretion density [numbers/g faeces]}}$$

The indicator organisms give a gross overestimation of the faecal input if the amounts of faecal sterols are used as a "true value." The use of *E. coli* would lead to an overestimation of the faecal load by more than three orders of magnitude and the use of enterococci by more than two orders of magnitude. In an example of QMRA for greywater (see section 3.6.1), coprostanol was used as a conservative biomarker.

The pathogen density in the untreated greywater can be calculated subsequently. Naturally, a higher faecal load may prevail in other circumstances and the figures adjusted accordingly:

$$\frac{(0.04\ [\text{g per person per day}] \times \text{excretion density [numbers/g faeces]} \times \text{excretion time [days]} \times \text{yearly incidence})}{(64\,900\ [\text{ml/day}] \times 365\ [\text{days}])}$$

with the faecal load, excretion density and excretion time expressed as probability density functions.

Sediment is formed in several in-house piping installations and can provide growth niches for bacteria, including indicator bacteria and pathogens, such as *Salmonella* and *Campylobacter* introduced from poor food handling. *Campylobacter* die rapidly from the effects of temperature, competition from commensal microbiota and nutrient unavailability (Ottosson & Stenström, 2003b). *Campylobacter* isolates of clinical importance are not likely to grow at temperatures below 30 °C (Hazeleger et al., 1998) and will not regrow under conditions common in greywater treatment systems. *Salmonella* can grow at 20 °C and below but is likely to be suppressed by the indigenous microorganisms, as shown by Sidhu et al. (2001). The growth rate of *Salmonella* at 20 °C, 0.022 ± 0.02 log/day, was used in the worst-case scenario in further risk assessment calculations. In most situations, pathogens are likely to decline outside their host. Decay rates in sediment and other matrices used in QMRA are listed in Table 3.8. Enterococci can be used as a conservative index organism for *Salmonella* and *Campylobacter*; somatic coliphages and F-specific RNA bacteriophages for rotavirus; and spores of sulfite-reducing anaerobic bacteria for *Giardia* and *Cryptosporidium* (oo)cysts.

Table 3.7 Faecal indicators in a greywater system and the corresponding faecal load with an average flow of 64.9 litres per person per day

Organism/biomarker	Mean	Min	Max	Excretion density (log numbers/100 ml or mg/g faeces)	Mean faecal load (min–max) (g/person per day)
Coliform bacteria	8.1	5.5	8.7		
E. coli	6.0	4.3	6.8	10^{7} [a]	65 (1.3–410)
Enterococci	4.4	3.0	5.1	$10^{6.5}$ [a]	5.2 (0.2–26)
Sulfite-reducing anaerobes	3.3	2.3	4.8		
Somatic coliphages	3.3	1.4	4.0		
Coprostanol (µg/l)	8.6	3.1	14.9	12.74[b]	0.04 (0.016–0.076)
Cholesterol (µg/l)	17.3	7.4	31.6	5.08[b]	0.22 (0.094–0.40)

Min = minimum; max = maximum
[a] Geldreich (1978).
[b] Leeming, Nichols & Ashbolt (1998).

3.4 Survival in soils and on crops

Treatment of excreta should aim to fully or substantially eliminate pathogens before their application as a fertilizer. Nevertheless, in practice, inactivation of pathogens in the soil may contribute importantly to overall risk reduction. Inactivation is often more rapid in the soil and on crop surfaces than in stored excreta and greywater and more rapid on crops than in soils. Some pathogens can persist, however, for extended periods of time in soil or on crop surfaces and can be transmitted to humans or animals. The most environmentally resistant pathogens are helminth eggs, which in extreme cases can survive for several years in the soil. In Volume 2 of the Guidelines, the background evidence for pathogen survival in soils and crops, which also applies to excreta and greywater, has been reviewed. A summary of this information is included in this section.

Pathogen inactivation is much more rapid in hot and/or sunny weather than under cool, cloudy or rainy conditions. The persistence in cold temperatures is relevant for post-harvest storage. The greatest health risks are associated with insufficiently treated excreta in combination with crops eaten raw — for example, salad crops, root crops (e.g. radish, onion) or crops grown close to the soil (e.g. squash). Certain crops may be more susceptible to contamination than others — for example, onions (Blumenthal et al., 2003), squash (Armon et al., 2002) and lettuce (Solomon, Yaron & Matthews, 2002). The surface properties of certain crops (e.g. hairy, sticky, with

Table 3.8 Decay rate of selected microorganisms in different matrices and at different temperatures[a]

Microorganism	Decay rate (log/day)	Matrix	Temperature (°C)	Method	Reference
Bacteria					
Salmonella typhimurium	−0.048 ± 0.0092	Greywater sediment	4	Culture	Ottosson & Stenström (2003b)
	−0.12 ± 0.0011		20		
	−0.36	Greywater	ambient		Nolde (1999)
Campylobacter jejuni	−1.30 ± 0.16	River water with sediment	25	Culture	Thomas, Hill & Mabey (1999)
	−0.11 ± <0.01		15		
	−0.02 ± <0.01		5		
Enterococci (bacterial indicator)	−0.032 ± 0.016	Greywater sediment	4	ISO 7899-2	Ottosson & Stenström (2003b)
	−0.078 ± 0.038		20		
Viruses					
Rotavirus	−0.016 ± 0.010	Liquid waste	12–17	Cell culture	Pesaro, Sorg & Metzler (1995)
	−0.119 ± 0.00835[b]	Grass	4–16		Badawy, Rose & Gerba (1990)
ΦX174 bacteriophage (viral indicator)	−0.018 ± 0.0048	Sediment	4	ISO 10705-2	Ottosson & Stenström (2003b)
	−0.11 ± 0.031		20		
MS2 bacteriophage (viral indicator)	−0.021 ± 0.0069	Sediment	4–20	ISO 10705-1	Ottosson & Stenström (2003b)
	−0.029 ± 0.024	Groundwater	4	Plaque assay	Yates, Gerba & Kelley (1985)
Parasites					
Cryptosporidium parvum oocysts	−0.006 ± 0.031	River water	15	Excystation	Medema, Bahar & Schets (1997)
	−0.010 ± 0.032		5		
	−0.011 ± 0.008		15	Dye exclusion	
	−0.010 ± 0.016		5		
Giardia intestinalis cysts	−0.042	Water	25	Dye exclusion	Romig (1990)
Spores of sulfite-reducing anaerobes (parasite indicator)	−0.00045 ± 0.0027	Sediment	4–20	ISO 6461/2	Ottosson & Stenström (2003b)
	−0.027 ± 0.0043	River water	15	Culture	Medema, Bahar & Schets (1997)
	−0.012 ± 0.0031		5		

[a] Values other than for greywater were used as reference values.

[b] Per hour.

crevices, rough, etc.) protect pathogens from exposure to radiation and make them more difficult to wash off. Crops that retain water (e.g. from rain, which, moreover, splashes up contaminated soil) are important in determining human exposure to pathogens. Lettuce retains a measured 10.8 ml of irrigation water, while a cucumber holds only 0.36 ml (Shuval, Lampert & Fattal, 1997). Stine et al. (2005) showed that lettuce and cantaloupe surfaces retained pathogens from irrigation water spiked with *E. coli* and a bacteriophage (PRD1), but bell peppers, which are smooth, did not.

Information on bacterial reduction is often based on *E. coli* as an index organism or includes information about the frequency of detection of pathogens such as *Salmonella* spp. on the crops. These values may be used in extrapolation of the risks and generally provide validation that high amounts of these bacterial groups will be reduced below a background level within 1–2 weeks or what is found on market products if irrigated with treated wastewater (Armon et al., 1994; Bastos & Mara, 1995; Vaz da Costa Vargas, Bastos & Mara, 1996). A withholding time of at least one month between application of treated excreta and harvest is recommended in these Guidelines (which partly lowers the risk related to wastewater irrigation). Recommended levels of $<10^3$ *E. coli* per gram total solids or $<10^5$ *E. coli* in greywater would be appropriate (see chapter 4).

Petterson, Teunis & Ashbolt (2001) modelled the inactivation of enteric viruses on lettuce and carrots using data collected on crops grown under greenhouse conditions with a model virus *Bacteroides fragilis* B40-8. Initial die-off was rapid, but a more persistent subpopulation of viruses survived throughout the experiment. Ward & Irving (1987) observed survival times of 1–13 days when the irrigation water contained between 5.1×10^2 and 2.6×10^5 type 1 poliovirus VU/l (decimal reduction needed to be useful in risk assessment). Petterson & Ashbolt (2003) summarized viral die-off data on different crops. These data are expressed as T_{99} values (number of days required for a two-logarithm reduction), not exceeding four days for leaf crops and 20 days for root crops. A withholding time of one month would normally ensure a safety margin against viral and bacterial contamination alike. On lettuce spiked with *Cryptosporidium* oocysts, no viable oocysts were detected after three days at 20 °C, while 10% remained at 4 °C (Warnes & Keevil, 2003). The inactivation rate is often considered to be more rapid on crops than in soils, with T_{90} values in the range of a few days (Asano et al., 1992; Petterson, Ashbolt & Sharma, 2001). Studies carried out in greenhouses in the United Kingdom (Stott et al., 1994) with seeded effluent (*Ascaridia galli*) indicated that irrigation with wastewater containing 10 eggs per litre resulted in low levels of nematode contamination on lettuce (maximum of 1.5 eggs per plant), and improving wastewater quality further to ≤ 1 egg per litre resulted in very slight contamination of only a few plants (0.3 egg per plant). These values correspond with the excreta target values, with the exception that the latter will give less contamination of the plant surfaces. The accidental occurrence of a few viable eggs can, however, never be excluded and, due to the latency period, may represent a potential risk to consumers in relation to both wastewater (see Volume 2 of the Guidelines) and excreta use. Data on pathogen survival in soil and on different crops are presented in Tables 3.9 and 3.10.

3.5 Epidemiological and risk-based evidence

Epidemiological evidence in relation to the reuse of treated excreta and greywater in agriculture is generally lacking. In areas where untreated human excreta are used as a fertilizer for crops, an elevated prevalence of *Ascaris* infection has occasionally been reported (Iran: Arfaa & Ghadirian, 1977; China: Xu et al., 1995). Hookworm infection

Table 3.9 Estimated survival times and decimal reduction values of pathogens during storage of faeces and in soil

Microorganism	Survival at 20–30 °C (days)[a]		Time needed for 90% inactivation of pathogen (T_{90}) at ~20 °C (days)[a]		Absolute max[d]/ normal max survival in soil[e]
	Faeces and sludge[b]	Soil[b]	Faeces[c]	Soil[c]	
Bacteria					1 year / 2 months
Thermotolerant coliforms	<90, usually <50	<70, usually <20	*E. coli*: 15–35	*E. coli*: 15–70	
Salmonella	<60, usually <30	<70, usually <20	10–50	15–35	
Viruses	<100, usually <20	<100, usually <20	rotavirus: 20–100 hepatitis A: 20–50	rotavirus: 5–30 hepatitis A: 10–50	1 year / 3 months
Protozoa (*Entamoeba*)	<30, usually <15[f]	<20, usually <10[e]	*Giardia*: 5–50 *Crypto-sporidium*: 20–120	*Giardia*: 5–20 *Crypto-sporidium*: 30–400	? / 2 months
Helminths (eggs)	Several months	Several months	*Ascaris*: 50–200	*Ascaris*: 15–100	7 years / 2 years

?, unknown; max, maximum

[a] Estimated survival times and decimal reduction values of pathogens during storage of faeces and in soil; presented in days if not stated otherwise.

[b] Feachem et al. (1983).

[c] Schönning et al. (in press).

[d] Absolute maximum for survival is possible under unusual circumstances, such as at constantly low temperatures or under well protected conditions (Feachem et al., 1983).

[e] Kowal (1985).

[f] Data are missing for *Giardia* and *Cryptosporidium*; their cysts and oocysts might survive longer than presented here for protozoa (Feachem et al., 1983).

is also prevalent in wet climates when excreta are used (Viet Nam: Needham et al., 1998; China: Xu et al., 1995). Blum & Feachem (1985) include descriptive studies of the prevalence of helminth infections in areas where untreated excreta are used as fertilizer. The risks to consumers and farm workers exposed to untreated or treated excreta used as fertilizer for crops, mainly from older studies, are shown in Table 3.11. The examples indicate that exposure to treated nightsoil was significantly associated with a reduction in *Ascaris* and hookworm infection compared with exposure to untreated nightsoil. Baseline prevalence rates in the study groups were similar.

A more recent study from Viet Nam focused on the traditional treatment of faeces before use as fertilizer (Humphries et al., 1997). Women helped prepare and distribute the faeces on the crops. Most used fresh faeces, but some used wet, dry or composted faeces for fertilizer. Dry faeces mixed with ash were distributed with a shovel or by hand, whereas wet faeces were mixed with water and poured onto the plants using

Table 3.10 Survival of various organisms on crops at 20–30 °C

Organism	Survival on crops (days)
Viruses	
Enteroviruses[a]	<60 but usually <15
Bacteria	
Thermotolerant coliforms	<30 but usually <15
Salmonella spp.	<30 but usually <15
Shigella spp.	<10 but usually <5
Vibrio cholerae	<5 but usually <2
Protozoan cysts	
Entamoeba histolytica cysts	<10 but usually <2
Cryptosporidium oocysts	<3 but usually <2
Helminths	
Ascaris eggs	<60 but usually <30
Tapeworm eggs	<60 but usually <30

[a] Poliovirus, echovirus and coxsackievirus.
Sources: Feachem et al. (1983); Strauss (1985); Robertson, Campbell & Smith (1992); Jenkins et al. (2002); Warnes & Keevil (2003).

dippers or buckets. Treatment of faeces consisted of mixing dry faeces with ash and putting the mixture in a pit along with coconut and banana leaves and organic waste. Most families used the faeces before it had been stored for four months (Hanoi Medical School, unpublished observations, 1994). Women who reported using fresh faeces as fertilizer had significantly higher hookworm egg counts ($P < 0.05$) than women who used treated faeces or who did not use human faeces as fertilizer. Since the results were not reported separately for those who used treated faeces, a conclusion about the effectiveness of treatment of faeces on hookworm infection cannot be drawn. There is some indication, from the data presented, that treatment of faeces may reduce the number of women with higher-intensity infections. The epidemiological study showed that the use of fresh faeces as fertilizer was associated with increased intensity of hookworm infection when compared with the use of treated faeces or no use of excreta as fertilizer. Comparisons are lacking between those who used treated faeces and those who did not use excreta. Excreta treatment before use or other management procedures to reduce risk should always be advocated. Treatment with ovicide could be considered (as occurs in parts of China), along with consideration of technologies for dry excreta storage and composting or thermophilic digestion.

Comparisons can be made with epidemiological studies on the use of raw wastewater. These have revealed an increased risk of parasitic and other enteric infections associated with raw wastewater use in agricultural irrigation (Katzenelson, Buium & Shuval, 1976; Fattal et al., 1986; Cifuentes, 1998; Srikanth & Naik, 2004; see also Volume 2 of the Guidelines). Several foodborne outbreaks of disease have been associated with the irrigation of crops with sewage-impacted water (Colley, 1996; Hardy, 1999; Doller et al., 2002) The treatment options for wastewater (e.g. in storage lagoons) seem to be efficient in reducing the transmission of pathogens and are also relevant for greywater use (Shuval, 1991; Blumenthal et al., 2001).

Table 3.11 Studies of risks to consumers and workers exposed to untreated or treated excreta in agriculture: prevalence of parasitic infections in exposed versus non-exposed populations[a]

Health outcome	Excreta quality	Population group	Prevalence of infection or reinfection after treatment (%)	Relative risk	Study group and comparison	Reference
Ascaris	Overflowing septic tank contents and excreta composted with animal manure	School children	(i) 14.3 vs 2.9 (ii) 6.7 vs 2.9	(i) 4.9[b] (ii) 2.3	School children (i) in urban area where vegetables fertilized with overflowing septic tank contents vs in sewered urban area; (ii) in rural area where human faeces composted with animal manure or applied at "appropriate" time to vegetables vs in sewered urban area	Anders (1952)
Ascaris	Untreated	Farming population	52 vs 0	52.0[b]	Families using excreta as garden fertilizer vs families using animal manure as garden fertilizer	Harmsen (1953)
Ascaris (positive conversion after chemotherapy)	Ovicide treated	Farming population	(i) 27.4 vs 41.5 (ii) 35.9 vs 41.5	(i) 0.66 (0.51–0.86)[c]** (ii) 0.86 (0.69–1.07)	(i) Ovicide-treated nightsoil vs untreated nightsoil (ii) Ovicide-treated nightsoil (commercial preparation) vs untreated nightsoil	Kozai (1962)
(i) *Ascaris* (prevalence)	Ovicide treated	Farming population	(i) A: 11.0 vs 17.5 B: 21.0 vs 33.1 C: 14.6 vs 11.6	(i) A: 0.63 (0.40–0.98)[c]* B: 0.63 (0.44–0.92)* C: 0.79 (0.53–1.18)	(i) A: After nightsoil treatment with ovicide plus chemotherapy vs before treatment B: After nightsoil treatment with ovicide vs before treatment C: Chemotherapy alone	Kutsumi (1969)
(ii) *Trichuris* (prevalence)			(ii) 47.1 vs 65.0	(ii) 0.73 (0.64–0.82)	(ii) After nightsoil treatment plus ovicide vs before treatment	

Table 3.11 (continued)

Health outcome	Excreta quality	Population group	Prevalence of infection or reinfection after treatment (%)	Relative risk	Study group and comparison	Reference
Hookworm (positive conversion after chemotherapy)	Ovicide treated	Farming population	(i) 17.7 vs 32.2	(i) 0.55 (0.36–0.81)[c]**	(i) Ovicide-treated nightsoil vs untreated nightsoil	Kozai (1962)
			(ii) 17.4 vs 32.2	(ii) 0.54 (0.36–0.81)**	(ii) Ovicide-treated nightsoil (commercial preparation) vs untreated nightsoil	
Hookworm (positive conversion after chemotherapy)	Ovicide treated	Adults	7.1 vs 12.5	0.56 (0.27–1.16)	Families using ovicide-treated nightsoil vs untreated nightsoil	Kutsumi (1969)
Hookworm	Treatment with ash and storage	Adult women		$P < 0.05$	Egg counts in women using fresh faeces vs women using treated faeces or not using faeces as fertilizer	Humphries et al (1997)

[a] Comparison is exposed vs unexposed for untreated excreta use; comparison is treated vs untreated excreta or after vs before treatment for treated excreta.
[b] Crude relative risk calculated from prevalence or incidence data reported.
[c] Relative risk and 95% confidence interval calculated from prevalence or incidence rates and population data reported. Statistical significance at levels $P < 0.05$ (*) and $P < 0.01$ (**).

3.6 Quantitative microbial risk analysis

Use of excreta and greywater in agriculture is currently practised mainly at the household and community levels and to a lesser extent as part of overall large-scale management schemes. In both levels of application, it is necessary to ensure realistic protection, which is a reflection of exposure and the disease prevalence in a given area. A key objective of urine collection and use is to minimize faecal cross-contamination. The same applies for greywater. Thus, the baseline in assessing both these types of systems is the degree of faecal contamination. The general recommendation for urine storage is mainly aimed at reducing the microbial health risks from consuming urine-fertilized crops. It will also reduce the risk for persons handling and applying the urine. In greywater use systems, the main objective is to minimize contact with the untreated greywater in larger systems as well as in small-scale applications. Subsurface wetlands as well as resorption systems will minimize contact. Greywater treatment in pond systems will reduce the content of potential pathogens present. In relation to guideline values, it is essential to consider the phenomenon of overestimating the health risks due to regrowth of indicators. Elevated indicator values should therefore always be assessed in relation to potential faecal inputs.

In one large-scale collection system for source-separated urine, the faecal cross-contamination was estimated to be within a range of 1.6–18.5 mg of faeces per litre of urine, with a mean of 9.1 ± 5.6 mg/l, thus resulting in about a 5 log lower concentration of potential pathogens in urine than in faeces. The faecal contamination of greywater was at a similar level, estimated to correspond to a faecal load of 0.04 g per person per day. These values were based on a relationship with levels of coprostanol measured. Comparing these levels with the amounts occurring in wastewater, they correspond to a conservative risk level that is at least 1000-fold lower than for wastewater. Using this relationship, a combination of treatment and other management options would need to achieve a 2.9 (maximum) or 1.6 (minimum) log reduction for protozoa and a 3.3 (maximum) or 2.3 (minimum) log reduction for viruses in urine and greywater to reach a 10^{-6} DALY median annual risk per person based on the total exposure volume. For faeces, however, the corresponding values would be about 5 logs higher.

The performance targets that apply to guarantee a technological safety and barrier effect against microbial hazards should ensure that the collection and handling of excreta and greywater are done so as to minimize exposure to untreated material, even if the relative risks are substantially lower in urine and greywater. Small communities have limited capacity and capability to run individual system assessment and management plans. Therefore, competent authorities should support the necessary implementation of system assessment and management plans and should function as reference points (see further institutional aspects in chapter 10). Performance targets assist in the selection and use of control measures that are capable of preventing pathogens from breaching the technical and handling barriers. In addition, they should minimize overall exposure to untreated excreta. Simple design, handling practices and exposure control are crucial.

3.6.1 Example of risk calculation for a greywater scenario

In greywater systems, microbial hazards emanate mainly from faecal cross-contamination (e.g. from anal cleansing, hygienic practices, contaminated laundry and other sources). Pathogens may also be introduced through food preparation.

Exposure to potential pathogens in greywater may occur through direct contact, contaminated drinking-water sources and groundwater recharge where the exposure depends on drinking-water treatment. Greywater used for irrigation may, depending on distribution practices, expose people via inhalation of aerosols as well as through consumption of irrigated contaminated crops, in a similar pathway as for wastewater (see Volume 2 of these Guidelines).

Ottosson (2003) made a risk calculation for a greywater system with pretreatment in a settling tank and activated sludge step before the water entered a pond system. The reference organisms chosen were *Salmonella*, *Campylobacter*, rotavirus and the parasitic protozoa *Giardia* and *Cryptosporidium*. The performance of the treatment steps was assessed and modelled for treatment barrier efficiency. The assessed barriers and transmission pathways are summarized in Table 3.12.

The faecal load in the greywater in the system was assessed based on a range of microbial indicators (*E. coli*, enterococci, sulfite-reducing clostridia, coliphages) and chemical markers (faecal sterols). The faecal input to the greywater was estimated to be 0.04 ± 0.02 g faeces per person per day from the quantification of the faecal sterol coprostanol, compared with 65 g and 5.2 g per person per day using *E. coli* or enterococci as indicators (see Table 3.13).

Table 3.12 Transmission pathways for exposures to used or discharged greywater and health-related modelling units involved, except treatment

Exposure	Health-related modelling units involved	Volume ingested
1) Drinking recharged groundwater (yearly risk from 365 exposures)	Dilution,[a] unsaturated zone[a] and saturated zone	$e^{(6.87 \pm 0.53)}$ ml/day[b]
2) Accidental ingestion of treated greywater (one-time exposure)	Pond	1 ml/exposure
3) Ingestion from a field irrigated with treated greywater (yearly risk from 26 exposures)	Survival on grass	1 ml/exposure
4) Ingestion/inhalation of aerosols	Tank	$e^{(-4.2 \pm 2.2)}$ ml[c,d]
5) Swimming in recreational water receiving treated greywater	Dilution	$e^{(3.9 \pm 0.3)}$ ml
6) Untreated greywater, *Salmonella* regrowth	Sink trap (growth)[e]	0.1 g

[a] Asano et al. (1992).
[b] Roseberry & Burmaster (1992).
[c] Dowd et al. (2000).
[d] Kincaid, Solomon & Oliphant (1996).
[e] Ottoson & Stenström (2003b).

Table 3.13 Indicator occurrence, measured as excreted organisms per person per day, and the corresponding faecal load in greywater (flow 64.9 litres per person per day)

Organism	Indicators in greywater	Excretion rate (per gram of faeces)	Faecal load (g per person per day)
E. coli	$10^{8.8}$ cfu	10^{7} cfu	65
Faecal enterococci	$10^{7.2}$ cfu	$10^{6.5}$ cfu	5.4
Coprostanol	0.56 mg	12.74 mg	0.04

Source: Ottosson & Stenström (2003a).

E. coli and enterococci may grow on the easily degradable organics in greywater. Their use as indicators for faecal load would therefore result in overestimation in the order of 1000 and 100 times, respectively. In the QMRA, coprostanol was used as a conservative biomarker.

Decay rates were based on either available information for the organism in question or enterococci as the indicator organism for *Salmonella* and *Campylobacter*, somatic and F-specific bacteriophages for rotavirus and spores of sulfite-reducing anaerobic bacteria for *Giardia* and *Cryptosporidium* (oo)cysts.

Four exposure scenarios were validated for the applied risk estimates in the QMRA:

1) accidental ingestion of 1 ml treated greywater, pond outlet (P_{out});
2) accidental ingestion of 1 ml treated greywater, pond inlet (P_{in});
3) yearly risk from direct exposure after irrigation with greywater, assuming 1 ml intake per day, 26 days a year;
4) yearly risk from drinking groundwater recharged from the pond as described in Asano et al. (1992), with modifications on the environmental die-off data and the water intake.

The different approaches used were as follows:

1) measuring faecal contamination in greywater with coprostanol concentrations and using epidemiological data to assess risks, as in Höglund, Ashbolt & Stenström (2002);
2) using a dose–response model derived from occurrence of faecal enterococci in marine waters (Kay et al., 1994), assuming an exponential probability of infection;
3) using faecal enterococci as indicator organisms for the presence of *Salmonella* in greywater based on sediment experiments.

In all exposure scenarios, rotavirus posed the highest risk, partly due to its excretion in higher numbers, at least during the acute phase, compared with the other pathogens included in the study. *Giardia* cysts and *Cryptosporidium* oocysts have low infectious doses but were not excreted in sufficient amounts to constitute a substantial health risk with the low faecal load registered. A shift upwards will naturally occur with higher faecal loads, anticipated in other types of setting. The average number of (oo)cysts in untreated greywater was simulated as approximately 0.002 (oo)cysts/ml, compared with 1.7 rotavirus particles/ml. Ottosson & Stenström (2003a) suggested that guidelines for the safe use of greywater in agriculture should not be based on thermotolerant coliforms as a hygienic parameter, because of the large input of non-faecal coliforms and/or growth of coliforms, unless their concentrations are adjusted for false-positive levels. The overestimation of the faecal load, and thus risk, resulting from these indicator bacteria is to some degree compensated for by the higher susceptibility to treatment and environmental die-off. The risk model based on faecal enterococci densities correlated well to the risk from viruses, which is supposed to be the most prominent in a system without disinfection due to their high excretion rates, environmental persistence and low infectious doses.

3.6.2 Example of risk calculation for collection and use of diverted human urine

The scenario considered for the urine diversion included the following transmission pathways (from Höglund, Ashbolt & Stenström, 2002):

1) ingestion of urine that has not been stored: workers may be accidentally exposed while cleaning blocked toilet drains, through ingestion in the case of splashing while emptying the collection tank or by contaminated hand-to-mouth contact;
2) ingestion of stored urine: farmers or other workers may accidentally ingest urine during handling of stored urine;
3) inhalation of aerosols while fertilizing crops with urine;
4) consumption of crops fertilized with urine.

The densities of pathogens are dependent on the prevalence of enteric diseases and the quantity of faeces that cross-contaminates the urine. For the collected urine, two different scenarios that will have an effect on pathways 2, 3 and 4 above were considered:

- *worst case scenario*: an epidemic had taken place right before the tank was emptied, resulting in no substantial inactivation in the collection tank;
- *sporadic case scenario*: the enteric disease events were evenly spread out during the time of collection (one year); thus, continuous inactivation occurred within the collection tank.

The risk calculations for stored urine considered the survival of microorganisms in urine (Höglund & Stenström, 1999; Höglund, Ashbolt & Stenström, 2002). The validations were performed at 4 °C and 20 °C. The effect of storing urine from one to six months was investigated in the QMRA.

The volume accidentally ingested was assumed to be 1 ml in pathways 1 and 2, as used for unintended ingestion of reclaimed wastewater (Asano et al., 1992).

For the inhalation of aerosols, the method of fertilizing crops is important. In large-scale applications, many farmers may use equipment (i.e. a splash plate) that spreads the urine approximately 1 m above the ground. In this case, the created drops are large (>1 mm) and will quickly settle. As a worst-case scenario, spray irrigation was assumed, and the risk for people living in the vicinity was calculated using a Gaussian plume model (Matthias, 1996). The resulting exposure will be 0.83 m^3 of aerosol per hour (Dowd et al., 2000) at a distance of 100 m from the point of spraying. No die-off of microorganisms was assumed to occur within the aerosol, which might be more conservative than reported (Mohr, 1991; Ijaz et al., 1994).

To assess microbial risks from crop ingestion, Shuval, Lampert & Fattal (1997) measured 10.8 ml of wastewater to attach to 100 g of lettuce, and Asano et al. (1992) assumed 10 ml to be ingested by consuming crops irrigated with wastewater. *Campylobacter jejuni*, *Cryptosporidium parvum* and rotavirus were chosen as indicator organisms. Pathogen probability density functions in urine were calculated from lognormal distributions of faecal cross-contamination, excretion days and excretion numbers (Table 3.14). The inactivation data were based on Asano et al. (1992) and Petterson, Teunis & Ashbolt (2001) and use of a uniform triangular distribution for rotavirus inactivation on crops (k-values recalculated to T_{90} values) during the period between fertilization and harvest. Since protozoa and bacteria reportedly have shorter survival times on crops than do viruses, the same T_{90} values were used as a conservative assumption for these microbial groups.

Table 3.14 Probability density functions used to calculate microbial health risks from various exposures to source-separated human urine

	C. jejuni	*C. parvum*	Rotavirus
Mean pathogen density (number per litre) (worst-case scenario)	4 564	152	243 793
T_{90} in urine, 4 °C (per day)	1	Triang(17, 29, 79)	No reduction
T_{90} in urine, 20 °C (per day)	1	5	Triang(15, 35, 42)
T_{90} on crop (per day)	Triang(1.4, 2.2, 3.0)	Triang(1.4, 2.2, 3.0)	Triang(1.4, 2.2, 3.0)
Dose–response model	β-Poisson $N_{50} = 896$, $\alpha = 0.145$	Exponential k = 238.6	β-Poisson $N_{50} = 5.6$, $\alpha = 0.265$

Range of 1.6–18.5 mg (mean 9.1 ± 5.6 mg) of faeces per litre cross-contaminated the separated urine. Triang = Triangular probability density functions; minimum, most likely and maximum given. T_{90} = time for 90% reduction in viable pathogen numbers.
Source: Höglund, Ashbolt & Stenström (2002).

Pathway 1: Risk from exposure to urine that has not been stored
The estimated risks of infection by the three indicator pathogens following accidental ingestion of 1 ml of unstored urine are illustrated in Figure 3.2. In the case of an epidemic, where no inactivation was assumed to occur in the collection tank, viruses may pose an unacceptably high risk, and bacteria pose a greater risk than protozoa. Similarly, for sporadic cases evenly spread out during the year, the risk of viral infection is the same as during an epidemic at 4 °C (probability of infection P_{inf} = 0.81), since very low inactivation of rotavirus occurs at this temperature, and slightly lower at 20 °C (P_{inf} = 0.55). In contrast, the risk for bacterial infection decreases significantly if sporadic rather than epidemic cases occur, since a large proportion of the added bacteria would die during collection at the two temperatures. For *Cryptosporidium*, the risk is approximately 1 log lower if there are sporadic instead of epidemic cases in the population connected to the tank, and the collection occurs at 4 °C ($P_{inf} = 3.1 \times 10^{-6}$). Collection at 20 °C decreases the risk another log ($P_{inf} = 4.5 \times 10^{-7}$).

Pathway 2: Risk from exposure to stored urine
Due to the inactivation of pathogens, risks associated with accidental contact decrease during storage. The exception was rotavirus during storage at 4 °C, which yields the same risk independent of storage time. The risk for *Campylobacter* infections was negligible after one month of storage at either 4 °C or 20 °C. If the urine is stored at 20 °C, the mean risk from *Cryptosporidium* is 4.7×10^{-11} after only one month, whereas if stored at 4 °C for one or six months, risks will be 1.1×10^{-5} and 2.8×10^{-9}, respectively. The risk for viral infection was much higher than the risk for protozoan infection, and inactivation was measured only in urine stored at 20 °C. After six months at 20 °C, the mean risk was estimated to be less than 10^{-4} (Figure 3.3).

Pathway 3: Risk from exposure to aerosols
The risk for infection through aerosols during the distribution of urine on arable land depended mainly on the urine storage time (Höglund, Ashbolt & Stenström, 2002). For people within an area of 100 m from the application of urine, the risks for bacterial and protozoan infections were low at any of the storage conditions. However, the risk for rotavirus infection was 0.72 for unstored urine or urine stored at 4 °C, if an epidemic was assumed. If the urine was stored for six months at 20 °C before fertilization, the mean estimated risk was reduced to 3.3×10^{-5}.

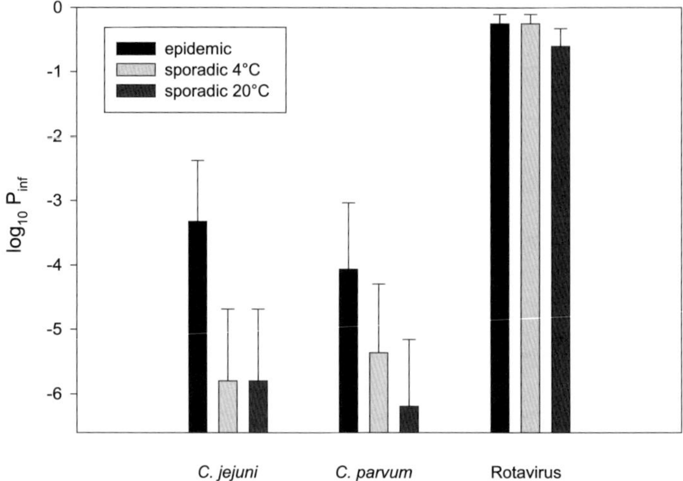

Figure 3.2
Mean probability of infection (5–95%) by *Campylobacter jejuni*, *Cryptosporidium parvum* and rotavirus following unintentional ingestion of 1 ml unstored urine for epidemic and sporadic scenarios and 4 °C or 20 °C during collection (Höglund, Ashbolt & Stenström, 2002)

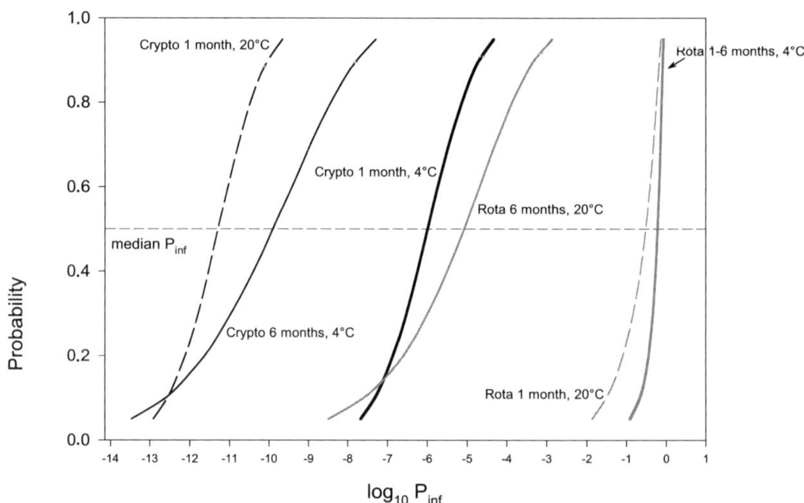

Figure 3.3
Probability of infection (5–95%) by *Cryptosporidium parvum* and rotavirus following ingestion of 1 ml stored urine (one or six months, 4 °C or 20 °C). *C. parvum* stored for six months at 20 °C yielded a risk that was $<10^{-15}$, as did *Campylobacter* after one month at both temperatures; this information has not been included in the figure (Höglund, Ashbolt & Stenström, 2000).

Pathway 4: Risk from exposure to fertilized crops

Possible risks following consumption of crops fertilized with fresh urine and urine stored for one or six months at 4 °C and 20 °C were examined. Crop withholding periods between one and four weeks were considered, to take into account the time between fertilization and crop consumption. The implications of different withholding periods following consumption of 100 g of raw crop fertilized with fresh urine are illustrated in Figure 3.4. With one week between fertilization and consumption, the risk for bacterial and protozoan infections was very low ($<10^{-5}$), whereas a three-week withholding period is needed for the risk of viral infection to reach the same level.

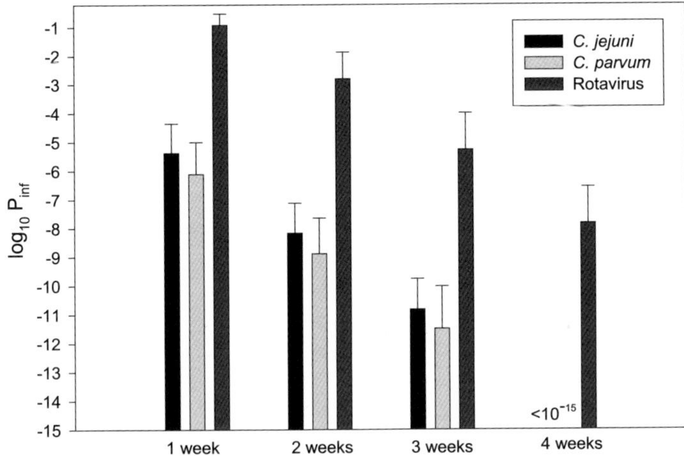

Figure 3.4
Mean probability of infection by pathogens following ingestion of crop fertilized with unstored urine with varying withholding periods. Error bars indicate one standard deviation (Höglund, Ashbolt & Stenström, 2002).

3.6.3 Example of risk calculation for stored but otherwise untreated excreta

A theoretical assessment was performed to evaluate risks for the transmission of infectious disease related to the local use of faeces as a fertilizer. The faeces were collected from dry urine-diverting toilets in single-family households and used in the household gardens. The faeces were treated only by means of storage in the temperature range up to 20 °C prior to the application. The pH was 6.7–8.4 and the dry matter content 20–40%. The material was not fully stabilized. The following five scenarios were evaluated:

1) application directly without storage;
2) application after storage for 6 months;
3) application after storage for 12 months;
4) application and incorporation after storage for 6 months;
5) application and incorporation after storage for 12 months.

Application means that the faeces were evenly distributed as topsoil, and incorporation means that the faeces were worked into the upper layer of the soil, resulting in a faeces to soil ratio of about 1:100.

Hazard identification

Organisms transmitted by the faecal–oral route were included, such as *Salmonella*, EHEC, rotavirus, hepatitis A virus, *Giardia*, *Cryptosporidium* and *Ascaris*.

Assessment of exposure
Each organism was modelled by probability density functions for incidence in the population, excretion and duration of infection, as well as die-off in the storage container and die-off in the soil after application of the material in the garden. Incidence was based on official reporting of incidence data for a European country adjusted for the underestimation (Wheeler et al., 1999). Using the resulting incidence, the probability that the faeces in the storage container from a typical household contained at least one type of pathogen was calculated to be 11.6%. The die-off of pathogens is based on collected information from both human faeces and other materials, such as animal manure and sewage sludge, to establish probability density functions for the inactivation. The human exposure was assumed to take place as accidental ingestion of small amounts of faeces or faeces and soil mixture during:

- emptying of the container and distribution of the material;
- recreational activities in the garden;
- gardening.

The faeces–soil intake was based on a literature study by Larsen (1998) in which children were estimated to ingest approximately 200 mg of soil per day on an average, with an absolute maximum of 5–10 g per day occurring once every 10 years through daily exposure. It was further assumed that adults ingest 15–50% of this amount, with a maximum of 100 mg per day. The container is emptied once a year, assuming that only adults are exposed.

Dose–response relationships
There is no information available on susceptible population subgroups, such as children, the elderly or immunocompromised, and as such it is not accounted for in the models. Less susceptible groups in the population were not accounted for either. The uncertainty of the parameters in the dose–response relationships was included.

Microbial risk calculation
Calculations were made for two main scenarios:

1) applying the incidence in the population (unconditional);
2) assuming that one member of the family actually had an infection during the period of collection (conditional).

The variations in the risk for infection depend on the organism in question. Some *Salmonella* are able to regrow in stored but unstabilized materials, especially if the materials are partly moist. Viruses and parasites generally have longer survival in the environment as well as lower infectious doses, which resulted in high risks for rotavirus, the protozoa and *Ascaris*. The difference in risk between the conditional and unconditional scenario was 1–4 orders of magnitude, and the difference between typical (50%) and worst case (95%) varied from none to five orders of magnitude, depending on the organism. For the unconditional scenario, the risk was never higher than 4×10^{-2} (rotavirus). Only after 12 months of storage and taking incidence into consideration were the risks $<10^{-4}$ for all organisms, excluding *Ascaris* ($P_{inf} = 8 \times 10^{-4}$), when emptying the container and applying the material.

In approximately 9 out of 10 gardens, the use of stored faeces as a fertilizer would not result in any risk of infection. Rotavirus and *Giardia* would be the most frequently occurring pathogens based on the incidence in the population. The die-off during storage would be substantial for, for example, *Salmonella*, while *Ascaris* in particular would have a much higher persistence in faeces. The pathogen with the most severe symptoms, EHEC, was reduced to very low levels during storage in the toilet and did not constitute any significant risk in any of the scenarios. Use of material directly after emptying the toilet container resulted in median risks exceeding those for the unconditional scenario with rotavirus and the parasites. After one year of storage, however, the median risks were below this level for all pathogens, as well as in the conditional scenario (i.e. a family member excreting the pathogen), with the exception of *Ascaris*. The worst-case risks, however, exceeded the level of 10^{-4} for viruses and parasites. The exposure to faeces in terms of ingested amounts was lower during recreational activities or gardening than when emptying the container due to the mixing with soil. Since the frequency of exposure was higher in the former exposure, however, the annual risks were almost as high.

4
HEALTH-BASED TARGETS

This chapter deals with health-based targets and related recommendations for health protection. The potential to relate protective measures that respond to health risks to guideline values or good practice is determined by the compliance level that can be expected realistically. It is less practical to apply guideline values in small-scale settings, where procedural and best practice guidance may offer a better approach.

An attempt has been made to harmonize the health-based targets presented in this volume with those in Volume 2 of the Guidelines (*Safe use of wastewater in agriculture*). Furthermore, issues specific to the safe use of excreta, urine and greywater in agriculture are pointed out. Obviously, the risk of transmission of pathogens through environmental pathways when unsanitized excreta are used in agriculture may lead to increased disease prevalence. Treatment of human excreta and other barriers against human exposure are considered the most important precautions against such transmission (see chapter 5).

Health-based targets need to be an integral part of the overall health policy, accounting for the trends in and relative importance of different transmission pathways, on both individual and household levels as well as in the overall management of public health. To ensure effective health protection, the target needs to be realistic, relevant to local conditions and commensurate with resources available for required protection methods. Health-based targets aim to improve public health outcomes and should support the rational selection of health safeguards, interventions and control measures, mainly in relation to excreta and greywater treatment, exposure control and safe handling.

The concept of health-based targets applies universally, irrespective of the level of development. Although the targets tend to be set at the national level, they are applied at the local level. Risks are subject to variability in performance of technical installations and the frequency of exposure. It is, therefore, necessary that recommendations be practical and take into account variability factors. Ad hoc events as well as behaviour may affect the health outcomes; thus, a "multiple-barrier approach" is needed.

The targets are part of an overall management and evaluation strategy in relation to health protection goals and implementation of the scheme to use excreta and greywater. In such contexts, any long-term effects also need to be considered. Where possible, the health-based targets should relate to quantitative risk assessment, taking into account local conditions and hazards. Epidemiological information on local handling and use of excreta and greywater in agriculture is scarce and scattered. The available epidemiological information on wastewater and sludge use can be partly applied in this context.

With increasing frequency, regulations and guidelines are based on the risk concept. By applying QMRAs, based partly on predictions and assumptions, sanitation systems can be evaluated and compared with established limits for acceptable risks. Treatment can also be adapted to reach a set of acceptable limits. Risk assessments can thus be made quite site specific, depending on information regarding, for example, the local health status of the population and behavioural patterns. An approach of setting acceptable local risk limits, applicable for sanitation systems where the use of the excreta products is practised, will relate to a subsequent change in the prevalence of infections. In developing countries with low sanitary standards, the goal will be to reduce the number of infections by implementing sanitation per se, including introducing new, more efficient treatment or exposure reduction alternatives, combined with other interventions related to safe treatment and storage, hygiene/health education as well as provision of access to safe drinking-water.

This volume of the Guidelines focuses on treatment, but also addresses other technical, practical and behavioural aspects intended to minimize the risk for disease transmission. Rules of thumb considered to obtain acceptable low risks are presented without a bias towards numeric limits in small-scale systems.

4.1 Type of targets applied

Health-based targets may be based on epidemiological evidence, risk assessment predictions, guideline values or performance. All have certain strengths and limitations. Health outcome targets based on epidemiological evidence are resource dependent and need a developed institutional verification system. Risk assessment targets are based on validated predictions but may overestimate the actual risks, due to variability in behaviour and exposure. Guideline values often have limitations in expressing the risks for a broad range of organisms. In many instances, performance targets based solely on indicator organisms have limitations in expressing the risks. They should preferably be based on a range of pathogens, considering their persistence under adverse treatment or environmental conditions. Performance targets should ensure that the performance assessment also reflects other, more vulnerable microbial groups and different conditions. All targets relate to variability and shorter periods of decreased efficiency in a number of processes. The targets should also reflect background rates of disease. Performance assessment does not normally need to be based on experimental evaluations carried out on site, but can be approximated using international evaluations that take the prevailing local conditions into account. It is, however, of value to put treatment performance evaluations in the hands of competent national or regional authorities or institutions. Different types of targets are summarized in Table 4.1 in relation to excreta and greywater use in agriculture.

In connection with the use of treated excreta and greywater, the health-based targets are related to exposure barriers and treatment performance in the overall risk assessment and risk management. Monitoring guideline values are mainly applicable in larger systems. The treatment alternatives give different levels of safety as barriers against pathogen transmission. Performance targets are further specified below, while the technical options and management aspects are dealt with in chapter 5. Numerical guideline values can be used mainly for validation, but should be applied with caution and always within a context of risk management strategies.

4.2 Tolerable burden of disease and health-based targets

The commonly accepted metric for expressing and comparing the burden of disease is the DALY (Murray & Acharya, 1997) (see also chapter 2). In the third edition of the *Guidelines for drinking-water quality* (WHO, 2004a), a tolerable burden of waterborne disease from drinking-water consumption of $\leq 10^{-6}$ DALY per person per year was adopted. This level can be compared with a microbial self-limiting diarrhoea and the corresponding case fatality rate of approximately 1×10^{-5} at an annual disease risk of 1 in 1000 (10^{-3}), which is also about 1×10^{-6} DALY (1 μDALY) per person per year (WHO, 2004a). Since food crops fertilized with treated excreta or irrigated with treated greywater, especially those eaten uncooked, are also expected to be as safe as drinking-water, the same high health protection level of $\leq 10^{-6}$ DALY per person per year is applicable in this context as well.

For operational purposes, treatment and other management options to reduce the level of pathogens and subsequently the degree of exposure should aim at this target.

Table 4.1 Nature, application and assessment of health-based targets

Type of targets	Nature of targets	Application	Assessment
Health outcome; epidemiology based	Reduction in detected disease incidence or prevalence	Microbial with high measurable disease burden Through direct impact measurement, such as food-associated disease	Public health surveillance; analytical epidemiology Often difficult to assess actual impact Multiple factors
Risk-based assessment	Tolerable level of risk due to direct or indirect exposure Relationship to other alternative use, exposure or sanitation facilities in local context	Microbial hazards in situations where disease burden cannot be directly measured	QMRA Predictive tool Needs to be related to local exposure
Quality targets	Guideline values	Measurements of pathogens or indicator organisms, less applicable in: - small-scale application - for urine due to rapid die-off of indicators - for greywater due to growth resulting in overestimation of risk	Measurements mainly valid in assessment of technical performance of treatment of faeces Should mainly be applied within a similar framework as for the assessment of wastewater use Ensure validity of measurement parameters (system validation) Limitations in reflecting general pathogen risks
Performance targets	Generic performance targets for removal of groups of organisms Customized targets Guideline values less applicable	Microbial contaminants	Compliance through system assessment Review by public health authorities Checklists Recommended for small-scale applications. Limitations based on local conditions
Specified technology	Authorities specify specific processes or system approaches to address constituent handling practices or behaviours in relation to health effects	Health effects in small-scale settings	Compliance assessment Operation and handling

Campylobacter, *Cryptosporidium* and rotaviruses were chosen as index organisms (Havelaar & Melse, 2003; WHO, 2004a). An example of a calculation of the values for tolerable infection risk is given in Volume 2 of these Guidelines and is also applicable in the context of this volume. The cited values accounting for the infection ratios are:

Rotavirus (industrialized countries)	1.4×10^{-3}
Rotavirus (developing countries)	7.7×10^{-4}
Campylobacter	3.1×10^{-4}
Cryptosporidium	2.2×10^{-3}

Thus, the tolerable disease risks for these organisms are in the range 10^{-3}–10^{-4} per person per year. This is a conservative value, given that the current global incidence of diarrhoeal disease in the age group 5–80+ is in the range 0.1–1 per person per year (see Volume 2 of these Guidelines).

Reliable epidemiological data relating to the safe use of excreta and greywater in agriculture are scarce. As an alternative, the range of tolerable disease risk can be deduced based on the QMRA, for which the risks resulting from exposure to faeces, urine and greywater were presented in chapter 3, for both its final use and handling. In this context, the current Guidelines are harmonized with the health aspects of the use of treated wastewater in agriculture, where the epidemiological appropriate level of tolerable risk for both crop consumers (unrestricted irrigation) and fieldworkers (restricted irrigation) has been identified (see Volume 2 of these Guidelines).

In chapter 5, the combination of different primary and secondary treatment barriers is described that can achieve a risk reduction to the health-based target level. Knowledge (or estimation) of the volume of treated excreta or greywater to which a person is exposed in the handling chain or that remains on the crop (ml or mg per 100 g crop) following fertilization, the withholding time and the die-off in the field will determine the degree of pathogen reduction required to achieve the tolerable additional disease burden of $\leq 10^{-6}$ DALY per person per year. This step requires the numbers of pathogens present in the untreated excreta or greywater to be known or estimated. In this context, the use of *E. coli* concentrations for verification monitoring is appropriate for treated excreta, but it is not for collected urine, due to a rapid die-off of the bacteria in this medium. In greywater, a regrowth of *E. coli* sometimes occurs, which may lead to an overestimation of the risks if verification monitoring is based on this parameter. It is suggested that *E. coli* guideline values, which are applicable for wastewater use, be applied cautiously for greywater. If applied, they will give a level of additional safety in this application, since the faecal load is usually 100–1000 times less than in wastewater. For helminth infections, the treatment verification monitoring level in terms of number of helminth eggs is presented in Table 4.2. The health-based protection to achieve the required pathogen reduction may consist of treatment alone or may be a combination of several measures. A guideline value of $<10^3$ *E. coli* per 100 ml is suggested for unrestricted irrigation with greywater. The target value of $<10^3$ *E. coli* per gram of treated faecal material applied as fertilizers would then ensure a comparative level of safety against bacterial pathogens and probably against viral pathogens as well. A clear value for parasitic protozoa does not exist.

The pathogen reduction that is needed in the on-site and off-site treatment of excreta is expressed as performance targets. This target for treated excreta is based on a storage time in the on-site treatment for 12–18 months of treatment (if only storage applies) and is combined with a stated withholding period that will further minimize

Table 4.2 Guideline values for verification monitoring in large-scale treatment systems of greywater, excreta and faecal sludge for use in agriculture

	Helminth eggs (number per gram total solids or per litre)	*E. coli* (number per 100 ml)
Treated faeces and faecal sludge	<1/g total solids	<1000/g total solids
Greywater for use in:		
• Restricted irrigation	<1/litre	$<10^5$ [a] Relaxed to $<10^6$ when exposure is limited or regrowth is likely
• Unrestricted irrigation of crops eaten raw	<1/litre	$<10^3$ Relaxed to $<10^4$ for high-growing leaf crops or drip irrigation

[a] These values are acceptable due to the high regrowth potential of *E. coli* and other faecal coliforms in greywater.

risks to the consumers. This period applies as the treated excreta are applied as a fertilizer and soil conditioner, which differs from the wastewater values, where the water is mainly used for irrigation purposes. The verification in relation to target values for *E. coli* and helminths is, however, applicable for faeces after storage/treatment.

Strauss & Blumenthal (1990) suggested that one year of storage was sufficient under tropical conditions (28–30 °C), whereas at lower average temperatures (17–20 °C) 18 months would be needed. Storage is especially beneficial in dry and hot climates where rapid desiccation of the material takes place and low moisture contents aid pathogen inactivation. Esrey et al. (1998) stated that there is rapid pathogen destruction at moisture levels below 25% and that this level should be aimed for in dry urine diversion toilets that are based on dehydration (i.e. storage). Low moisture content is also beneficial in order to reduce odour and fly breeding. Regrowth of bacterial indicators and some pathogens (EHEC and *Salmonella*) may, however, occur after application of moisture (water) or if the material is mixed with a moist soil, as indicated by results reported by Austin (2001).

The reduction of viruses in excreta is related to storage period and storage conditions. Figure 4.1 exemplifies this with a risk calculation for rotavirus in relation to storage.

Protozoan cysts are sensitive to desiccation, and this also affects their survival on plant surfaces (Snowdon, Cliver & Converse, 1989; Yates & Gerba, 1998). Normal moisture levels do not inactivate *Ascaris* eggs. Moisture levels below 5% are needed (Feachem et al., 1983), but information on the corresponding inactivation time is currently lacking.

To treat excreta, thermophilic digestion (50 °C for 14 days) and composting in aerated piles for one month at 55–60 °C (plus 2–4 months of further maturation) are recommended and generally accepted procedures that will satisfy the reduction of pathogens to achieve the health-based target values. Recommendations for treatment of, for example, faecal sludge and organic household waste (food waste) also rely on such temperatures (EC, 2000). Under controlled conditions, composting at 55–60 °C for 1–2 days is sufficient to kill essentially all pathogens (Haug, 1993). The longer periods stated give a handling margin. It is common that cold zones form within the digested or compost material, resulting in local areas with less inactivation.

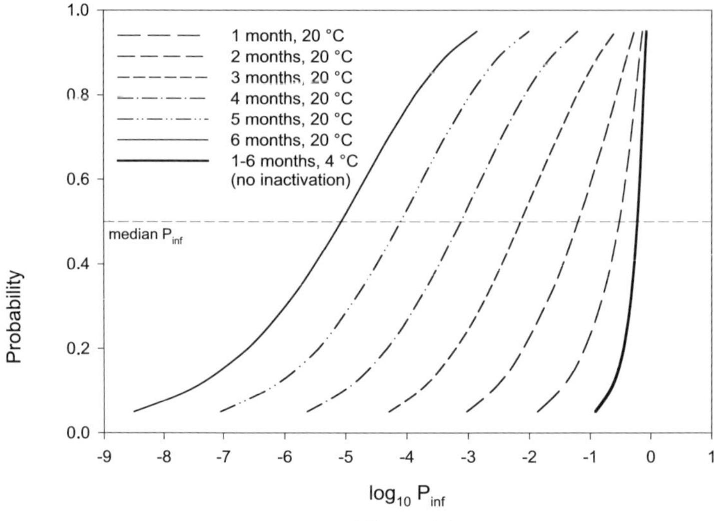

Figure 4.1
Effect of storage time on rotavirus risk (from Höglund, Ashbolt & Strenström, 2002)

4.3 Microbial reduction targets

The approach adopted in these Guidelines focuses on risks from the chain of excreta and greywater use from collection to the consumption of food crops eaten. Data on health effects were used to assess the infectious disease risk and harmonize with the approach taken in Volume 2 of the Guidelines. The analyses took account of consumption of crops eaten raw and of risks from direct contact with treated excreta (involving involuntary soil ingestion). Direct correlations between the relative risks of wastewater and treated excreta applications have not been established. However, the guideline values presented for both are in the same range as exemplified for *Ascaris* in Box 4.1.

Based on the exposure scenario for wastewater irrigation, it was shown that, in order to achieve $\leq 10^{-6}$ DALY per person per year for rotavirus, total pathogen reductions of 6 log units for the consumption of leaf crops (lettuce) and 7 log units for the consumption of root crops (onions) are required. Applying these values to excreta, this implies about an 8–9 log reduction for faeces (assuming a 100-fold dilution). The risk from source-separated urine and greywater relates to the faecal cross-contamination that occurs. Based on measurements, this cross-contamination is usually less than 10^{-4} of excreta, thus similar to a 100-fold dilution of wastewater with a need for a pathogen reduction of <4–5 log units as the performance target for unrestricted irrigation to achieve the tolerable additional disease burden of $\leq 10^{-6}$ DALY per person per year.

As an example, in source-separated urine, the faecal cross-contamination was estimated to be within a range of 1.6–18.5 mg of faeces per litre of urine, with a mean of 9.1 ± 5.6 mg/l, thus resulting in about a 5 log lower concentration of potential pathogens than in faeces. The faecal contamination of greywater was at a similar level, estimated to correspond to a faecal load of 0.04 g/person per day. Because the risks associated with exposure to rotavirus are estimated to be the highest, this level of

Box 4.1 Comparative performance targets for viable helminth eggs in wastewater, faecal matter and faecal sludge

- Wastewater performance target for unrestricted irrigation: ≤1 egg/litre
- Rw rate (water requirements expressed in m/year), compared with an egg application rate on the soil, Re, of: Re < 10^7 Rw (eggs/ha·year)

The use of treated excreta or faecal sludge should not enrich the soil with a higher egg concentration than the quantity permitted by the application of irrigation water. The sludge application rate depends on the egg concentration in the total solids Eg (expressed as eggs/g total solids). The sludge quantity applied to the soil Rs thus amounts to: Rs < Re/Eg = 10^7 Rw/Eg (g total solids/ha·year).zYearly helminth load from irrigation (using an average of, e.g., 500 mm/year): ≤500 helminth eggs/m^2·year permissible. Application of treated faecal matter (same quantities as in good agricultural practice of manure): 10 t manure/ha·year at 25% total solids (1 kg/m^2· year) = 250 g total solids/m^2·year.

[helminths eggs]tolerable ≤500/250 = 2 helminth eggs/g total solids
(with 1000 mm/year: 4 helminth eggs/g total solids)

Guideline value set to 1 helminth egg/g total solids (to account for variability).

pathogen reduction will provide sufficient protection against bacterial and protozoal infections.

These log unit pathogen reduction levels may be achieved by the application of appropriate health protection measures, each of which has its own associated log unit reduction or range of reductions (Table 4.3). A combination of these measures is used such that, for all combinations, the sum of the individual log unit reductions for each health protection measure adopted is equal to the required overall reduction. Several of the steps are similar to what has been presented in Volume 2 of the Guidelines, while the pathogen reduction due to treatment will differ. Treated excreta are always applied as a fertilizer in combination with planting or during the initial growth period. Thus, a withholding period of normally more than one month applies, except for application of greywater, which is normally done for irrigation purposes.

In Volume 2 of these Guidelines, it was stated that in order to achieve the health-based target of ≤10^{-6} DALY per person per year for rotavirus, wastewater treatment is required to reduce the *E. coli* count by 4 log units or a similar pathogen reduction. The corresponding reduction of raw faecal material will thus be 6 log units, while normally a 2 log unit reduction will suffice for urine and greywater.

Microbial reduction targets for protection against helminth infections are based on the results of microbiological studies. Although investigations related to risk should be based on the number of viable eggs, in the microbiological investigations, the reduction refers to the percentage of viable eggs out of the total egg population and not the actual numbers.

An effective health protection measure for removing helminth eggs from the surface of crops eaten uncooked (e.g. lettuce leaves) is washing the crop in a weak detergent solution (washing-up liquid is suitable) and rinsing thoroughly with safe drinking-water. Helminth eggs are very "sticky," so they easily adhere to crop surfaces; the detergent solution releases them into the aqueous phase. This control measure reduces the number of eggs on the crop surface by 1–2 log units (B. Jiménez-Cisneros, personal communication, 2005).

Table 4.3 Pathogen reductions achievable by various health protection measures

Control measure[a]	Pathogen reduction (log units)	Notes
Excreta storage without fresh additions	6	The required pathogen reduction to be achieved by excreta treatment refers to the stated storage times and conditions in Tables 4.4–4.6 (below) without addition of fresh untreated excreta (faeces and urine) as based on measurements and risk calculations. Pathogen reductions for different treatment options are presented in chapter 5, and examples of risk calculations in chapter 3.
Greywater treatment	1–>4	Values relate to the treatment options described in chapter 5. Generally, the highest exposure reduction is related to subsurface irrigation.
Localized (drip) irrigation with urine (high-growing crops)	2–4	Crops, where the harvested parts are not in contact with the soil.
Materials directly worked into the soil	1	Should be done at the time when faeces or urine is applied as a fertilizer.
Pathogen die-off (withholding time one month)	4–>6	A die-off of 0.5–2 log units per day is cited for wastewater irrigation. The reduction values cited here are more conservative to account for a slower die-off of a fraction of the remaining organisms. The log unit reduction achieved depends on climate (temperature, sunlight intensity, humidity), time, crop type and other factors.
Produce washing with water	1	Washing salad crops, vegetables and fruit with clean water.
Produce disinfection	2	Washing salad crops, vegetables and fruit with a weak disinfectant solution and rinsing with clean water.
Produce peeling	2	Fruits, root crops.
Produce cooking	6–7	Immersion in boiling or close-to-boiling water until the food is cooked ensures pathogen destruction.

Sources: Beuchat (1998); Petterson & Ashbolt (2003); NRMMC & EPHCA (2005).

Treatment processes to achieve, or partially achieve, the pathogen reductions exist. Different investigations show that in collected and stored dry faecal material, a time period of between 6 and 12 months may suffice with the application of an elevated pH and high ambient temperature (Table 4.4 and Table 4.5). If the number of helminth eggs is ≤1 per g total solids, then no additional health protection measures are required in relation to this group of organisms, as the target value is automatically achieved (this is the typical situation in most industrialized countries).

4.4 Verification monitoring

To ensure that health-based targets are being met, it is important to develop performance targets that can be monitored. There are three types of monitoring:

- Validation is the initial testing to prove that a system as a whole and its individual components are capable of meeting the performance targets and, thus, the health-based targets.

- Operational monitoring is the routine monitoring of parameters that can be measured rapidly (i.e. through tests that can be performed quickly, parameters measured online, or through visual inspection) to inform management decisions to prevent hazardous conditions from arising.
- Verification monitoring is done periodically to show that the system is working as intended. This type of monitoring usually requires more complicated or time-consuming tests that look at parameters such as bacterial indicators (*E. coli*) or helminth eggs.

Monitoring is further discussed in chapter 6. Verification monitoring requirements for treated faecal sludge, urine and greywater are discussed below.

4.4.1 Treatment of excreta and greywater

Pathogen numbers in raw or treated faecal sludge, excreta or greywater are not measured routinely (if at all). The performance of the on-site treatment used to partially or wholly ensure $\leq 10^{-6}$ DALY per person per year cannot, therefore, be determined on the basis of pathogen verification monitoring, but instead is based on validation of the general treatment efficiency. Verification monitoring is applicable mainly in larger collection systems or when a secondary off-site treatment after collection from a number of individual units is made. The microbiological performance of the larger system or the off-site treatment is evaluated by determining the content of a pathogen indicator bacterium, such as *E. coli*, in the treated material. The same applies for larger greywater collection and treatment systems, where the effluent may be monitored for verification purposes. For large-scale systems or when secondary off-site treatment is necessary, the values in Table 4.2 above apply.

When other exposure barriers are appropriate and can be enforced, the above guideline values can be relaxed based on national or local decisions — for example, when a public body has the legal authority to require that crop restrictions be followed regularly or when a strong project management exists. For fruits and vegetables, special restrictions may apply. For subsurface adsorption systems for greywater, no guideline values apply. However, the siting of such systems should not interfere with groundwater quality. For pond systems for greywater treatment, the risk of promoting mosquito breeding should be evaluated, and pond systems should not be opted for under circumstances where vector breeding may have a substantial impact on health without incorporating mosquito control measures into their design and operation.

4.4.2 Other health protection measures

Operational health protection measures include the agricultural use practices and the preceding treatment and transport. Even if a treatment is validated and verification monitoring has been done, process steps or handling practices may periodically malfunction, resulting in a fertilizer product that is not completely safe. Therefore, additional measures should be taken in order to further minimize the risk for disease transmission. These measures are applicable independent of the scale of the system (special considerations for small systems are provided in section 4.4.3). Thus:

- Excreta and faecal sludge should be treated before they are used as fertilizer, and the treatment methods should be validated.
- Equipment used for, for example, transportation of unsanitized faeces should not be used for the treated (sanitized) product.

- Precautions related to the handling of potentially infectious material should be taken when applying faeces to soil. These precautions include personal protection and hygiene, including hand washing.
- Treated excreta and faecal sludge should be worked into the soil as soon as possible and should not be left on the soil surface.
- Improperly sanitized excreta or faecal sludge should not be used for vegetables, fruits or root crops that will be consumed raw, excluding fruit trees.
- A withholding period applies for treated excreta and faecal sludge. This period should be at least one month.
- The treatments given in Table 4.4 can be used as off-site secondary treatment (material removed from toilet and primary treatment at the household level).

Table 4.4 Additional treatments for excreta and faecal sludge off-site, at collection and treatment stations from large-scale systems (municipal level)[a]

Treatment	Criteria	Comment
Alkaline treatment	pH >9 during >6 months	Temperature >35 °C and/or moisture <25%. Lower pH and/or wetter material will prolong the elimination time.
Composting	Temperature >50 °C for >1 week	Minimum requirement. Longer time needed if temperature requirement cannot be ensured.
Incineration	Fully incinerated (<10% carbon in ash)	

[a] Run in batch mode without addition of new material.

Composting is recommended mainly as an off-site secondary treatment at a large scale, since the process may be difficult to run. Temperatures above 50 °C should be obtained in all material for at least one week. Times may need to be modified based on local conditions. Large systems need a higher level of protection than what is required at the household level, and additional storage adds to safety. Storage at ambient conditions is less safe, but acceptable, if the conditions above apply. Shorter storage times can be applied for all systems in very dry climates where a moisture level below 20% is achieved. Sun drying or exposure to temperatures above 45 °C will substantially reduce the time required. Rewetting may result in growth of *Salmonella* and *E. coli*.

4.4.3 Excreta in small systems

For smaller systems, validation together with operational monitoring apply. In small-scale systems in developing countries, it is impractical or even impossible to relate performance to actual guideline values. Validation of dry collection of excreta from latrines in Viet Nam showed that it is possible to achieve a total die-off of *Ascaris* ova and indicator viruses (>7 log reduction) within a six-month period (mean temperature 31–37 °C, pH 8.5–10.3 in the faecal material and moisture content 24–55%) (Carlander & Westrell, 1999; Chien et al., 2001). At lower temperatures (approximately 20 °C), longer storage times apply for a total destruction of *Ascaris* (Phi et al., 2004), although similar high reductions were found under cold conditions in China (Wang, 1999; Lan et al., 2001). Addition of a pH-elevating chemical (e.g. lime or ash) has been shown to enhance the inactivation of pathogens in small systems. Other methods to reduce the pathogen content rely on elevation in temperature, desiccation or prolonged storage at ambient conditions.

The practical options depend on the scale of the system (i.e. at household or municipal level). More technical options are available at the municipal scale. Implementation of treatment on an individual level has added difficulties, involving people's (often well established) habits and practices. The scale also influences the combinations of suitable primary and secondary treatments and barriers. Handling systems need to be adapted to the different treatments. Within operational monitoring, the on-site storage conditions given in Table 4.5 apply.

Table 4.5 Recommendations for storage treatment of dry excreta and faecal sludge before use at the household and municipal levels[a]

Treatment	Criteria	Comment
Storage; ambient temperature 2–20 °C	1.5–2 years	Will eliminate bacterial pathogens; regrowth of *E. coli* and *Salmonella* may be considered if rewetted; will reduce viruses and parasitic protozoa below risk levels. Some soil-borne ova may persist in low numbers.
Storage; ambient temperature >20–35 °C	>1 year	Substantial to total inactivation of viruses, bacteria and protozoa; inactivation of schistosome eggs (<1 month); inactivation of nematode (roundworm) eggs, e.g. hookworm (*Ancylostoma*/*Necator*) and whipworm (*Trichuris*); survival of a certain percentage (10–30%) of *Ascaris* eggs (≥4 months), while a more or less complete inactivation of *Ascaris* eggs will occur within 1 year (Strauss, 1985).
Alkaline treatment	pH >9 during >6 months	If temperature >35 °C and moisture <25%, lower pH and/or wetter material will prolong the time for absolute elimination.

[a] No addition of new material.

For operational verification, the following points should further be considered for on-site storage and collection:

- Primary treatment (in the toilet) includes storage and alkaline treatment by addition of ash or lime.
- pH elevation to above 9 is preferred, which can be obtained by the addition of alkaline material (e.g. lime or ash; 200–500 ml; enough to cover the fresh faeces) after each defecation. (Total elimination may not occur, but a substantial reduction will be achieved.)
- Secondary off-site treatments as for larger systems (municipal level), including alkaline treatments, composting or incineration (Table 4.5), can be applied off-site and result in a further reduction when municipal collection is organized.
- In small-scale systems (household level), the faeces can be used after primary on-site treatment if the criteria in Table 4.3 are fulfilled.

As for larger collection and application systems, the following points need consideration:

- Personal protection equipment should be used when handling and applying faeces.
- Faeces should additionally be mixed into the soil in such a way that they are well covered.
- A withholding period of one month should be applied, i.e. one month should pass between fertilization and harvest.

4.4.4 Operational monitoring for urine in large- and small-scale systems

The major risks in relation to collected urine relate to faecal cross-contamination in the source-separating toilets. Specific recommendations for large-scale systems may need to be adapted based on local conditions, accounting for behavioural factors and the technical systems selected. If a system is clearly mismanaged (i.e. faeces can be seen in the urine bowl or other routes of cross-contamination are observed), prolonged storage should be applied. The recommended storage times related to pathogen reduction at different temperatures are based on validation monitoring and risk assessment calculations (Höglund, Ashbolt & Stenström, 2002). The operational verification is divided between larger systems with a central collection and family-based systems (Table 4.6). These values are applicable for all systems where the collected urine is mixed between several individual units and subsequently used as a fertilizer for crops.

For an individual one-family system and when the urine is used solely for fertilization on individual plots, no storage is needed.

Table 4.6 Recommended guideline storage times for urine mixture[a] based on estimated pathogen content[b] and recommended crop for larger systems[c]

Storage temperature (°C)	Storage time	Possible pathogens in the urine mixture after storage	Recommended crops
4	≥1 month	Viruses, protozoa	Food and fodder crops that are to be processed
4	≥6 months	Viruses	Food crops that are to be processed, fodder crops[d]
20	≥1 month	Viruses	Food crops that are to be processed, fodder crops[d]
20	≥6 months	Probably none	All crops[e]

[a] Urine or urine and water. When diluted, it is assumed that the urine mixture has at least pH 8.8 and a nitrogen concentration of at least 1 g/l.

[b] Gram-positive bacteria and spore-forming bacteria are not included in the underlying risk assessments, but are not normally recognized as causing any of the infections of concern.

[c] A larger system in this case is a system where the urine mixture is used to fertilize crops that will be consumed by individuals other than members of the household from which the urine was collected.

[d] Not grasslands for production of fodder.

[e] For food crops that are consumed raw, it is recommended that the urine be applied at least one month before harvesting and that it be incorporated into the ground if the edible parts grow above the soil surface.

Sources: Adapted from Jönsson et al. (2000); Höglund (2001).

During storage, the urine should be contained in a sealed tank or container. This prevents humans and animals from coming in contact with the urine and hinders evaporation of ammonia, decreasing the risk of odour and loss of nitrogen. The urine should preferably not be diluted. Concentrated urine provides a harsher environment for microorganisms, increases the die-off rate of pathogens and prevents breeding of mosquitoes; thus, the less water that dilutes the urine, the better.

Specific recommendations include the following:

- For vegetables, fruits and root crops consumed raw, a one-month withholding period should always be applied.
- In areas where *Schistosoma haematobium* is endemic, urine should not be used near freshwater bodies.

- Urine should be applied close to the ground and preferably mixed with or watered into the soil.

General recommendations for the use of urine are as follows:

- Direct use after collection or a short storage time is acceptable at the single household level.
- For larger systems, urine should be stored for times and under conditions given in Table 4.6.
- An interval of at least one month should be observed between fertilization and harvest.
- Additional stricter recommendations may apply on a local level, in the case of frequent faecal cross-contamination. The recommendations for storage times are directly linked to agricultural use and choice of crop (Table 4.6).

Additional practices to minimize the risks include the following:

- When applying the urine, precautions related to the handling of potentially infectious material should be taken. These precautions could, inter alia, include wearing gloves and thorough hand washing.
- The urine should be applied using close-to-the-ground fertilizing techniques, avoiding aerosol formation.
- The urine should be incorporated into the soil. This is best done mechanically or by subsequent application of irrigation water.

5
HEALTH PROTECTION MEASURES

On-site sanitation installations are likely to grow in numbers, and their use and performance are essential to achieve the targets for tolerable disease burden. Growing quantities of excreta and greywater will have to be dealt with. The excreta from these systems (i.e. from private and public toilets and from septic tanks) as well as the greywater from households are, in most cases, still disposed of untreated. Sanitation upgrading must not only aim at providing appropriate public and private facilities, but also facilitate the sustainable management of excreta and greywater, including collection, transport, treatment and use as fertilizer, soil conditioner, irrigation or for other purposes, such as surface water or groundwater recharge.

To achieve this, a combination of health protection measures needs to be taken that will produce overall pathogen reductions and that differ by system component. Pathogen reduction required for fresh excreta will be in the order of 2 log units higher than for wastewater (i.e. in the range of 8–9 log units), while pathogen reduction for source-separated urine and greywater will be substantially lower (i.e. about 3–5 log units), based on the measured faecal cross-contamination in these system components. Most of the health protection measures are similar to those for the safe use of wastewater (see Volume 2 of these Guidelines), but some fundamental differences exist — for example, the potentially higher concentration of pathogens in excreta and lower concentrations in urine and the substantially higher die-off that may be achieved in the field, since fertilization occurs mainly during planting and does not continue up to harvest. Otherwise, the control measures are similar and include:

- excreta and greywater treatment;
- crop restriction;
- proper excreta and greywater handling and application techniques;
- withholding periods for pathogen die-off between fertilization and consumption;
- appropriate food preparation measures (washing, disinfecting, peeling, cooking);
- human exposure control and hygiene education.

In planning for or assessing sanitation systems and health protection measures, it is of prime importance to take all components — e.g. sanitation facilities (toilets and latrines at private and public levels), treatment facilities, pit emptying, collection, transport — into consideration to the extent possible.

Health risks associated with excreta and greywater use are linked mainly to occupational exposure of those who handle the excreta and greywater and consumption of potentially contaminated products. Technology alone is unable to interrupt disease transmission and accompanying ill health, if hygiene awareness in a community is low. Poor domestic and personal hygiene diminish the positive impact of improved excreta and greywater management on community health. Treatment needs to fulfil a reliable reduction of different groups of pathogens so that the waste meets the quality guideline values and performance criteria. If this is achieved, disease transmission to those collecting and using the material as fertilizers as well as those consuming fertilized products will be reduced to acceptable levels.

Measures that prevent pathogens from reaching the agricultural produce and the selection of appropriate crops for fertilization (e.g. bioenergy crops or crops aimed for further processing) may prevent pathogens from affecting the consumer while taking advantage of the positive nutritional benefit of reliable fertilizers.

The feasibility and efficacy of any combination of health protection measures will depend on local factors, such as:

- availability of resources (e.g. fertilizers);
- existing social and agricultural practices;
- demand for fertilized food and non-food crops;
- existing patterns of excreta-related disease;
- health education and possibilities to ensure the efficacy of selected health protection and control measures.

Especially for greywater use, secondary risks may arise from the creation of habitats conducive to the breeding of insect vectors of disease and a subsequent increase in the transmission of vector-borne diseases. Conducting an analysis of the storage, treatment and irrigation options will identify the key risk points as a basis for the selection and design of the most appropriate health protection measures.

5.1 Specific considerations for exposure control in the use of urine, faeces and greywater

Treatment of excreta (faeces) can be either on-site directly in the toilet (e.g. by prolonged storage without mixing with untreated material, drying the material or the addition of a pH-elevating compound) or off-site, where the material is collected from the toilet and treated in a controlled way with the purpose of reducing pathogens to acceptable limits. Systems designed for primary on-site treatment will produce an initial pathogen die-off that can be further corrected through off-site treatment should monitoring reveal that the initial pathogen reduction is insufficient. This combination is optimal for health protection.

If secondary off-site excreta treatment is needed to reduce the risks to an acceptable level but is logistically not feasible, some of the other health protection measures should be deployed; for example, suitable crop restriction can make any further measures redundant. If the effective implementation and enforcement of crop restrictions are somehow not possible, then recourse to other measures will be necessary. Decision-making on measures should ensure that their deployment is progressive, incremental and synergistic. Small-scale use schemes for excreta and greywater are often subsistence-level operations that are difficult to control in relation to treatment efficiency. Measures often need to be developed for minimization of risks to the individual, including health education and improved access to safe domestic water supplies. It is often desirable to combine several health protection measures. For example, crop restriction may be sufficient to protect consumers but will need to be supplemented by additional measures to protect collectors or workers. Sometimes, partial treatment to a less demanding standard may be sufficient if combined with other measures.

Use of excreta and greywater is currently practised mainly at household and community levels and, only to a lesser extent, as part of overall large-scale management schemes. It is necessary to ensure realistic protection in all applications. The health-based targets should account for the exposure and the disease prevalence within a given area. A key objective of urine collection and use is to minimize faecal cross-contamination. The same applies for greywater. Thus, the baseline in assessing both these types of systems is the degree of faecal contamination that occurs. The general recommendation of urine storage is mainly aimed at reducing the microbial health risks from consuming urine-fertilized crops. It will also reduce the risk for persons handling and applying the urine. In greywater use systems, the main objective is to minimize contact with the untreated greywater in larger systems as well as in small-scale applications. Subsurface wetlands and resorption systems will minimize contact. Greywater treatment in pond systems will reduce the content of any pathogens present. In relation to guideline values, it is essential to consider the phenomenon of overestimating the health risks due to regrowth of indicators. Elevated indicator values should therefore always be assessed in relation to potential faecal input.

5.1.1 Exposure control: general principles

A systematic survey of a local system can identify potential risk factors and suggest ways to avoid pathogen exposure, either by reducing contact with the material or by implementing measures to decrease the number of pathogens in the material that will be handled. Reducing contact includes factors such as closed systems and ensuring adequate storage times, wearing personal protection, using proper handling tools and reducing contact in the field by working the excreta into the soil. General handling precautions are often defined as additional measures and not as proper barriers.

Treatment of excreta could be related to containment directly in the toilet in relation to defecation (e.g. by additives that will enhance the die-off of pathogens or prolonged storage) or by further treatment off-site in a controlled way with the purpose of reducing pathogen concentrations to acceptable limits. Esrey et al. (1998) stated that a combination of safe storage and fast destruction of the pathogens in excreta is needed in order to prevent contamination of the environment.

Inactivation of pathogens will also occur on agricultural land after application of the excreta as fertilizer and on crops that may have become contaminated by the application of fertilizer during crop development or from splashes from the soil during heavy rains. This inactivation over time depends on prevailing environmental conditions and functions as an additional barrier against exposure from handling and consumption of crops and for humans and animals entering the fertilized field. The additional reduction with time, constituting a "barrier function in agriculture," is of additional importance, especially for crops that are to be consumed raw. Also, for safe handling of other crops and reducing cross-contamination during food preparation, the withholding period (time between fertilization and harvest) is of importance.

In the use of treated excreta, urine or greywater, certain key risk points and exposure pathways need to be considered. These are elaborated below in this chapter. Furthermore, the risks are related to the degree of faecal cross-contamination of untreated faeces as well as the efficiency of treatment. The factors in Table 5.1 apply for most systems, but are of major concern in larger systems where several units or users are involved. Handling is further discussed in section 5.2.2.

This chain of events can be further illustrated with the example of faecal sludge emptying and use as a fertilizer in agriculture (Figure 5.1; Strauss et al., 2003).

5.1.2 Exposure control at agricultural sites or site of use

Exposure control related to the field and the use of products relates to (1) crop restriction, (2) application techniques, (3) fieldworkers, (4) the withholding period (period between fertilization and harvest) and (5) die-off of organisms before consumption. This section essentially follows the messages given in Volume 2 of the WHO *Guidelines for the safe use of wastewater, excreta and greywater*, with slight modifications.

Table 5.1 Major exposure points for the reuse of excreta and greywater

Risk activity[a]	Major exposure route	Groups at risk	Risk management considerations
Emptying the collection chamber/vessel (1–4)	Contact	Entrepreneurs Residents Local communities	Provision of protective clothing and suitable equipment for persons involved Training Facility should optimize on-site treatment Design of facility and selection of technology to facilitate safe emptying Avoid spillage
Transportation (1–5)	Contact Secondary spread through equipment	Entrepreneurs Local communities	Avoid spillage Equipment not used for other purposes without proper disinfection/cleaning
Off-site secondary treatment facility (1–3) Ponds (5)	Contact (all) Vectors	Workers Nearby communities	Ensure treatment efficiency Protective clothing Facility should be fenced off Ensure no access for children Consider and minimize vector propagation Exclude recreational activity and consider vectors (5)
Application (1–3, 5)	Contact Inhalation	Entrepreneurs Farmers Local communities	Use "close to the ground application," work the material into the soil directly and cover Reduced access should be ensured if quality is not guaranteed; in such cases, applications to parks, football fields or where the public have access should be avoided Protective clothing for workers Minimum one month between application and harvest
Crops Harvest Processing Sale (1–5)	Consumption Handling	Consumers Workers Vendors	Crops eaten raw pose the most risk; industrial crops, biofuels or crops eaten only after cooking pose less risk Adequate protective clothing (gloves, shoes) Provide safe water in markets for washing and refreshing vegetables
Consumption (1–5)	Consumption	Consumers	Practising good personal, domestic and food hygiene Cooking food thoroughly

[a] (1) Dry collection; (2) Faecal sludge; (3) Wet systems; (4) Urine; (5) Greywater.

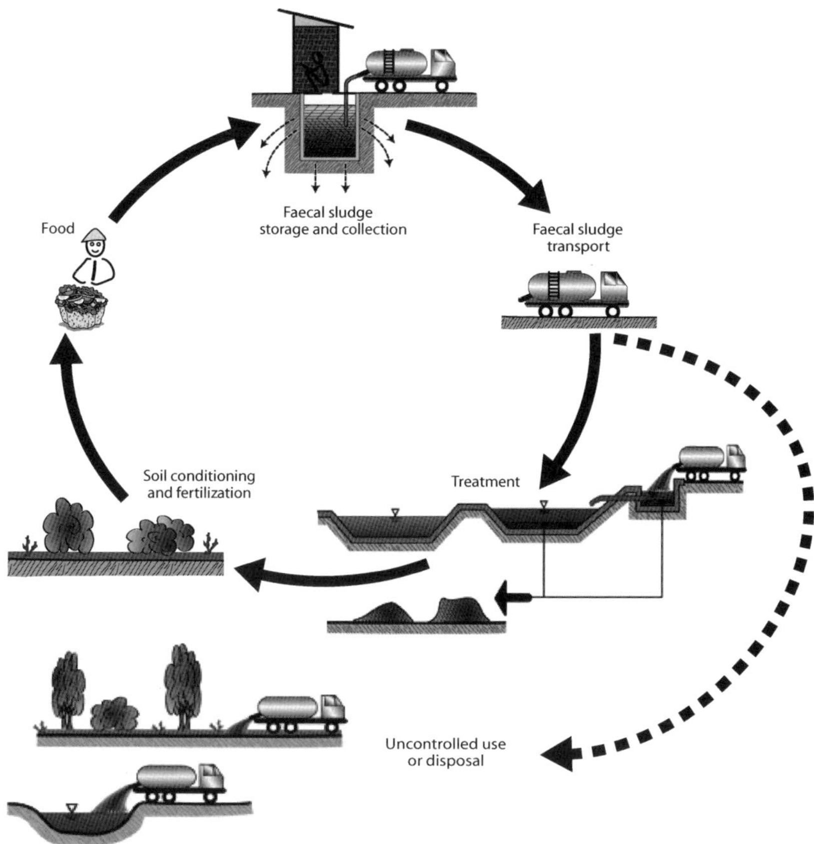

Figure 5.1
Critical control points in preventing enteric disease transmission in faecal sludge management

Crop restriction

Restricting crop selection does not normally need to be applied when treated urine and greywater are used, due to the low degree of faecal contamination. The use of treated excreta or faecal sludge may be restricted to non-food crops (e.g. cotton and bioenergy crops such as rapeseed or fast-growing woods, like *Salix* plantations used for biofuel). They may also be applied on crops processed before consumption (wheat) or crops that have to be cooked (potatoes). Crop restriction still requires that the excreta have been treated before use.

If greywater is heavily contaminated, vector breeding is likely to occur or pond treatment is not feasible, subsurface horizontal irrigation in the root zone of selected plants is a feasible option.

Application techniques

Irrigation with greywater and irrigation with wastewater share the same application techniques (see Volume 2 of the Guidelines). Localized irrigation with both greywater and urine is estimated to provide an additional pathogen reduction of 2–4 log units, depending on whether the harvested part of the crop is in contact with the soil or not (NRMMC & EPHCA, 2005). Urine should always be applied close to the ground and worked into the soil to minimize nitrogen losses; this also further reduces the risks. Treated excreta or faecal sludge can essentially follow the local practices applied for animal manure. The material should, however, be worked into the topsoil, both as a benefit for plant uptake and to reduce direct contact with any remaining pathogens.

Fieldworkers

Agricultural fieldworkers are at high potential risk, especially for parasitic infections. Treated human excreta are often applied on a small scale, which should result in less risk than indiscriminate open-air defecation. In larger-scale applications, such as the use of treated faecal sludge, exposure to helminth eggs can be eliminated or reduced by appropriate treatment combined with the use of appropriate protective clothing (e.g. shoes or boots for fieldworkers). These health protection measures have not been quantified in terms of pathogen exposure reduction, but they are expected to have an important positive effect. In larger-scale applications, fieldworkers should have access to adequate sanitation facilities and water for drinking and hygienic purposes. It is beneficial that effective hygiene promotion programmes targeting fieldworkers be linked to agricultural extension activities or other health programmes.

Withholding period

It is always recommended that there be a period of at least one month between application of urine or treated excreta or faecal sludge and crop harvesting. Vaz da Costa Vargas, Bastos & Mara (1996) showed that cessation of irrigation with wastewater for 1–2 weeks prior to harvest can be effective in reducing crop contamination by providing time for pathogen die-off. A further reduction will occur during a 30-day period. Risk calculations have been done for urine application to the field, showing that a withholding period of one month will result in a risk level much below 10^{-6} DALY for pathogenic bacteria, viruses and parasitic protozoa. Enforcing a withholding period for treated excreta is normally no problem, since the fertilizer is usually used at planting or applied on seedlings.

Die-off of organisms before consumption

The interval between final application of excreta as fertilizers and produce consumption reduces the number of pathogens substantially. In Volume 2 of the Guidelines, the study by Petterson & Ashbolt (2003) is cited, in which a substantial die-off is reported. The precise values depend on climatic conditions, with rapid pathogen die-off in hot, dry weather and less in cool or wet weather without much direct sunlight (approximately 0.5 log unit per day). With more conservative calculations, this reduction is at least 4 log units during a month and will give adequate safety when combined with other health protection measures. Helminth eggs can remain viable on crop surfaces for up to two months, although few survive beyond approximately 30 days (Strauss, 1996).

5.1.3 Post-harvest exposure control

Vigorous washing in tap water of rough-surfaced salad crops (e.g. lettuce, parsley) and vegetables eaten uncooked reduces bacteria by at least 1 log unit; for smooth-surfaced salad crops (e.g. cucumbers, tomatoes), the reduction is approximately 2 log units (Brackett, 1987; Beuchat, 1998; Lang, Harris & Beuchat, 2004). Washing in a disinfectant solution (commonly a hypochlorite solution) and rinsing in tap water can reduce pathogens by 1–2 log units. Washing in a detergent (e.g. washing-up liquid) solution and rinsing in tap water can reduce helminth egg numbers by 1–2 log units

(B. Jiménez-Cisneros, personal communication, 2005). Peeling fruits and root vegetables reduces pathogens by at least 2 log units. Cooking vegetables achieves an essentially complete reduction (5–6 log units) of pathogens.

These reductions are extremely reliable and should always be taken into account when selecting the combination of excreta/greywater treatment and other health-based control measures. Effective hygiene education and promotion programmes will be required to inform local food handlers (in markets, in the home and in restaurants and food kiosks) how and why they should wash produce fertilized with excreta and/or irrigated with greywater effectively with water or disinfectant and/or detergent solutions.

5.2 Technical measures

Excreta and greywater treatment and handling systems are often decentralized and involve no or limited sewerage. Currently available technology allows design of such systems in both urban and rural areas in rich and poor countries (Jenssen et al., 2004; Werner et al., 2004). In low-income countries, rural populations with access to sanitation facilities mostly use on-site installations such as traditional pit, ventilated improved pit (VIP) or pour-flush toilets and more recently, in selected areas, urine-diverting toilets. In contrast to the situation in industrialized countries, where the dominating urban sanitation system is centralized sewerage, the majority of urban dwellers in low- and middle-income countries are served by on-site sanitation systems. Small-diameter gravity sewers or other low-cost sewer systems might also prove feasible in selected, mainly densely populated urban areas served by reliable water supply. It is unlikely that sewerage will become a predominant sanitation option of choice in developing countries in the foreseeable future due to water scarcity and unreliability of water supply services and for financial, economic and resource reasons. Due to growing pressures on public health systems, environment and natural resources, a variety of reuse-oriented on- and off-site systems have been developed and implemented at an increasing rate (Werner et al., 2004). These comprise urine-diverting toilets, composting toilets, anaerobic (yielding biogas) and aerobic treatment of excreta and separate greywater treatment systems.

This section gives a brief overview of sanitation for low- as well as high-income countries where excreta and greywater are collected and treated for reuse in urban or periurban agriculture. This includes systems where excreta (urine and faeces diverted or combined) and greywater are handled separately and on site and cluster systems that handle combined wastewater through septic tanks and small-diameter sewers. Figure 5.2 summarizes some technical options for excreta and greywater management based on the collection, treatment and use options.

5.2.1 On-site sanitation systems

On-site sanitation systems serve a single home or small clusters of homes. They range from traditional septic tank or soil infiltration systems to the more recent source separating systems that are designed for recycling of resources from excreta and greywater (Figure 5.3). Systems where the excreta are treated and handled separately from the greywater are termed source separating systems, with either two fractions (the excreta — urine and faeces — and the greywater) or three fractions (urine, faeces and greywater).

Toilets that use no or very little water will limit collection to excreta only. The toilet options used in the source separating systems range from pit toilets to modern urine-diverting and vacuum toilet systems. The principal difference between the pit

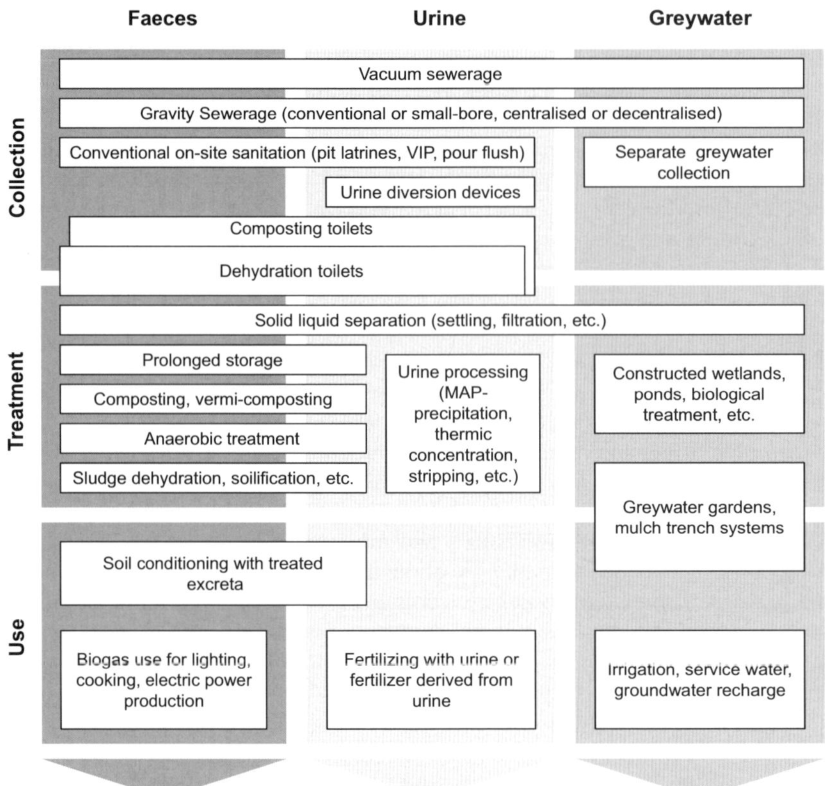

Figure 5.2
Overview of technologies for management of excreta and greywater

and pour flush toilets and the other options is that the former utilize pits or soak-aways in natural soils, which due to local soil and groundwater conditions may pose a threat to the groundwater quality and, therefore, to human health. The other options collect all excreta for on- or off-site treatment and potential use and thus provide better protection of the local groundwater. The pit toilets, constructed for disposal of excreta and not for use of the material, can also be excavated, providing possibilities of recycling of phosphorus and organic matter but losing nitrogen. The composting or dry sanitation toilets lose nitrogen to the air, while the urine-diverting or low-flush systems with holding tanks have very little loss of plant nutrients prior to agricultural application of excreta when they are handled properly. Greywater treatment options are described in section 5.2.4.

Pit toilets

Pit toilets include the simple pit latrine and VIP latrine, which do not require water for flushing, and pour flush toilets, where 1–3 litres of water are used to flush the excreta to a soak-away. Traditionally, pit latrines were dug quite deep, often discharging their percolate directly into groundwater. When pit latrines are used, shallow pits should be dug, since these may limit the groundwater impact as well as being easier to excavate for reuse after ample storage.

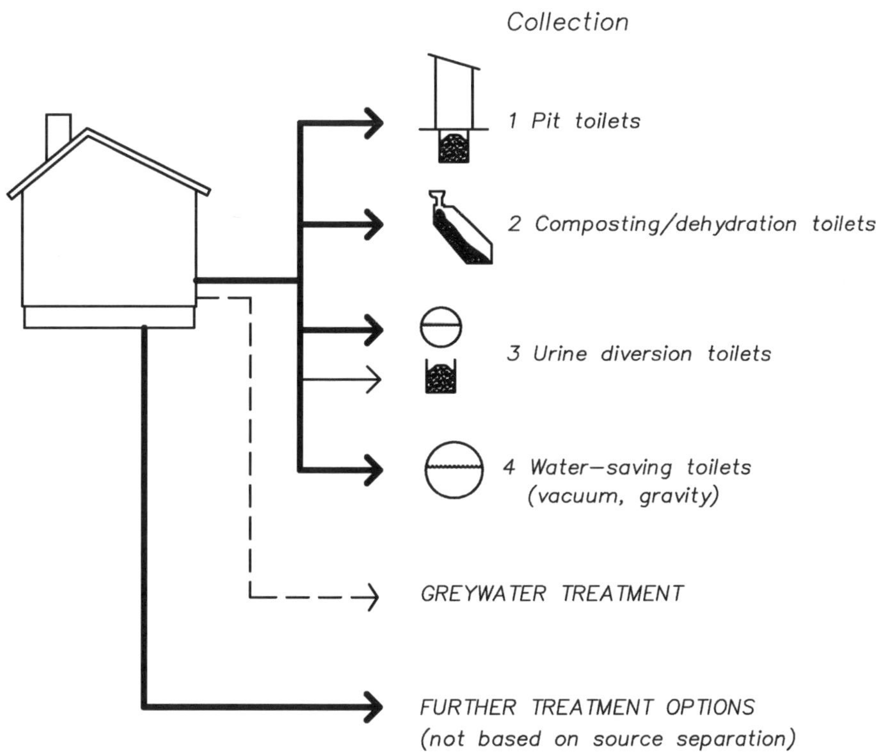

Figure 5.3
One-site sanitation options: 1-4, systems with source separation. For the systems with source separation, greywater is handled in a separate system (see section 5.2.4).

The separation distance between the latrine and the groundwater is an important hygienic barrier and should be maximized. It depends on several factors, such as the soil texture, structure, chemical composition and hydraulic loading. Normally, finer-grained soils (fine sand silt or finer) give better protection than coarser sands and gravel. Water use should be limited to anal cleansing and cleaning of the toilet. The toilet should be constructed so that no rain or surface water can flow into the pit, either when the toilet is in use or when the pit is full and covered for its contents to mature and sanitize.

The potential for fly breeding is reduced by a fly mesh at the ventilation pipe (VIP), the use of a toilet cover and frequent adding of bulking material or ash to reduce the possibility of flies coming into contact with fresh faecal material. Adding ash or lime will cause a rise the pH and enhance pathogen die-off.

When the pit is full, the waste should be covered with soil and the chamber sealed for two years. After two years of storage, the decomposed waste can be safely used as a soil addition (WHO, 1996).

Pour flush toilets use a pit for excreta disposal, have a special pan cast into the cover slab and are preferably also equipped with a water seal for odour and fly control. The pour flush toilets may be equipped with one or two soak-pits or discharge to septic tank systems (see below). Pour flush toilets are not suitable for areas with cold climates and impermeable or very low permeability soils (WHO, 1996). The potential risk for groundwater contamination is higher than for simple pit/VIP latrines due to the water use, and pour flush toilets should be avoided in areas of shallow water tables. Pour flush toilets are also inappropriate where the use of solid objects for anal cleansing (such as leafs, stones or corn cobs) is the custom, as these may cause siphon blockage.

Composting toilets

Composting toilets (Figure 5.4) have a collection chamber where all excreta are confined. Composting systems should preferably be operated in a batch mode, such as provided by the double vault system (B in Figure 5.4), where one vault is used while the other matures, or by collection containers (C in Figure 5.4), which are changed when full and set aside to mature and sanitize. This eliminates mixing of fresh and matured material and is safer for persons emptying the toilet. Secondary composting may be a way to ensure that material from composting toilets sanitizes properly. The toilets can be designed with or without urine diversion. Composting toilets rely mainly on aerobic degradation of organic matter, resulting in a volume reduction of the excreta of 70–90% if properly designed (Del Porto & Steinfeld, 1998). Adding dry bulking material is important; otherwise, it will not function as a composting toilet, but will be a collection chamber for wet excreta with potential odour and fly breeding problems. Proper ventilation will help improve odour control.

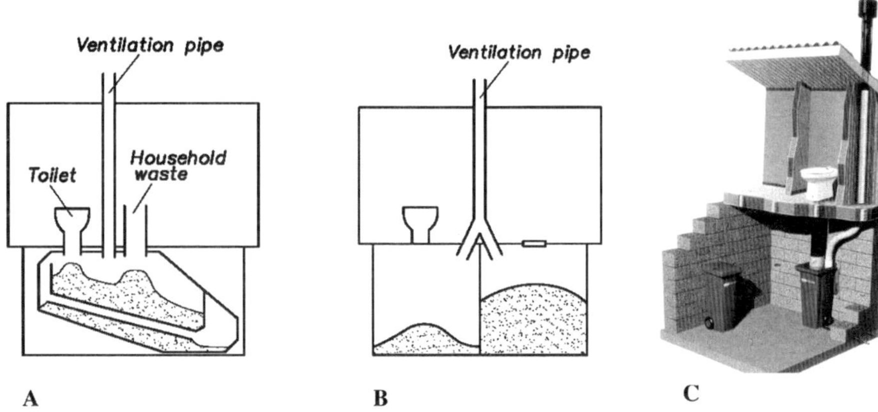

Figure 5.4
Examples of composting toilet systems: A, Continuous system; B, Batch system – dual compartment; and C, Batch system – removable compartments

The carbon to nitrogen ratio of excreta (including urine) is 7–8, but for well functioning composting it needs to be raised to between 30 and 35, which can be done by adding bulking material such as paper, wood or bark chips, sawdust, ash or other similar substances. The bulking material also serves to cover the fresh faeces and thus lower the potential for fly contact and breeding, reducing the risk of disease transmission. Adding bulking material also helps to mitigate odour problems. Organic household waste can also be added to a composting toilet through the toilet or through a separate chute (A in Figure 5.4). Adding organic household waste will help to raise the carbon to nitrogen ratio.

Thermophilic composting of faecal material normally gives a fast and substantial reduction of pathogens if elevated temperatures are reached. Experimentally, T_{90} values (i.e. 1 log reduction) are 6 min at 65 °C and 1 h at 52 °C for *E. coli*. Enterococci and viruses have a slower die-off rate (Eller, Norin & Stenström, 1996). Composting will fulfil the criterion of an acceptable risk reduction to below 10^{-4} per year (Watanabe Fan & Omura, 2002). Due to its complexity, however, the composting process may prove difficult to manage within the chamber. Experience from temperate regions has shown that it is difficult to reach temperatures above 40 °C in the composting compartment. The normal operating temperature range is therefore often mesophilic or ambient. Pathogen reduction may require either long maturation times or a secondary composting (section 5.2.3) or storage period.

Emptying composting toilets constitutes a critical handling point. Proper protection measures, mainly personal protection, should be taken if the material is not fully sanitized, and the material should be further treated or stored out of reach from people until proper maturation times have been reached. In addition to protective clothing (e.g. gloves and boots), normal hygiene and washing after the emptying operation are important (see also section 5.2.2 below).

Dehydration toilets

A dehydration toilet has the same basic construction as a composting toilet, with a collection chamber below the toilet. The aim, however, is to evaporate or dry out the excreta instead of optimizing the conditions for composting. In the dehydration toilet, the moisture content of the excreta is reduced. For efficient operation, neither water nor urine should be added to the dehydration chamber. With the aid of heat (preferably solar), natural evaporation, ventilation and the addition of absorbent materials, the moisture content is reduced and can be kept low. A combination of high temperatures and effective ventilation speeds up the desiccation process. Together with temperature and humidity, storage time and pH play important roles in the reduction of pathogens. The ventilation, which should draw air through the toilet and out through the vent pipe, as well as the absence of urine or other liquids help to reduce odours. This technology is increasingly popular in arid areas where water is scarce and faeces can be effectively dried and used as a safe fertilizer. After each defecation, absorbents such as lime, ash, sawdust or dry soil should be added to the chamber to absorb excess moisture and make the pile less compact. Addition of absorbents is also reported to reduce flies and eliminate bad odours. The use of alkaline absorbents, such as wood ash or lime, will result in an increase in pH of the pile and enhance pathogen die-off.

Several studies report the pathogen die-off rate in dehydrating toilets (Table 5.2). Early studies indicated that *Ascaris* eggs were particularly resilient to dehydration (Strauss & Blumenthal, 1990) but dependent on the temperature, moisture content and pH; 6–12 months in warm climates are usually sufficient to allow for the die-off of helminth eggs (Peasey, 2000). Investigations in Viet Nam have shown that a six-month retention period gave an 8 log reduction in resistant indicator viruses and no viable *Ascaris* eggs (Carlander & Westrell, 1999). The mean temperature ranged from 31 to 37 °C (overall maximum was 40 °C), the pH in the faecal material from 8.5 to 10.3 and the moisture content from 24% to 55%. The inactivation was described as a combination of factors, but pH for the virus indicator inactivation was shown to be statistically significant as a single factor (Carlander & Westrell, 1999; Chien et al., 2001). Another study indicated that a period of 12 months was needed to achieve a complete destruction of *Ascaris* eggs (Phi et al., 2004). In a Chinese study by Wang

(1999), plant ash was mixed with faeces in a ratio of 1:3 and yielded a pH of 9–10. A >7 log reduction in bacteriophages and faecal coliforms and a 99% reduction in *Ascaris* eggs were recorded after six months, even though the temperature was low (–10 to 10 °C), resulting in partial freezing of the material. Coal ash and soil addition led to a lower or insufficient reduction, respectively. The coal ash gave an initial pH of 8. Use of these additives warrants an extension of the subsequent storage time to 12–18 months without new faecal additions, and alternating collection chambers are recommended. According to Lan et al. (2001), a pH above 8 resulted in inactivation of *Ascaris* within 120 days.

Addition of a pH-elevating agent like lime or ash has the potential to enhance inactivation of pathogens. After alkaline treatment, the resulting fertilizer will have an elevated pH (>8). This may be beneficial for many soils, but it may affect crop production in already alkaline soils adversely. The conditions to achieve complete removal of pathogens may vary due to local circumstances. On a large scale, secondary treatment of collected material may function as an additional treatment

Table 5.2 Investigated microbial reduction in dry collection of faeces

Area of investigation	Type of toilet	Additive	pH, temperature, moisture	Most important findings: Inactivation of pathogens and indicators	Reference
Viet Nam (during hot and dry season)	12 latrines, 2 of each type; all urine-diverting, most double-vault or multi-bucket	Ash from firewood and leaves; 200–700 ml per visit	pH: 8.5–10.3 temperature: 31.1–37.2 °C moisture: 24–55% (mean values for each latrine)	**Controlled die-off experiments in challenge tests:** T_{90} for *Salmonella typhimurium* phage 28B varied from 2.4 to 21 days. pH most important factor for die-off. *Ascaris* viability 0–5% after 9 weeks (except in two latrines). pH in combination with temperature affect die-off.	Carlander & Westrell (1999)
South Africa (hot to cold climate)	Various urine-diverting toilets	Wood chips	pH: 8.6–9.4 moisture: 4–40%	**Organisms present in material:** After 10 months: All indicators present in high numbers (10^2–10^6/g). *Salmonella* present. After 12 more months: Faecal streptococci ~10^4/g, clostridia and coliphages present, *Salmonella* absent.	Austin (2001)
South Africa	2 urine-diverting toilets	Wood chips + turning	pH: 8.4–8.6 moisture: 4–9%	**Organisms present in material:** After 2 months: Indicators except coliphages present (~10^2/g). *Salmonella* absent.	Austin (2001)

Table 5.2 (continued)

Area of investigation	Type of toilet	Additive	pH, temperature, moisture	Most important findings: Inactivation of pathogens and indicators	Reference
El Salvador	118 double-vault urine-diverting latrines; 38 single-vault solar latrines	Lime, ash or lime-mixed soil	pH: 6.2–13.0	**Organisms present in material:** Faecal coliforms inactivated after 500 days. pH most important factor. *Ascaris* inactivated after 450 days (pH >11), after 700 days (pH 9–11). Temperature strongest predictor for inactivation.	Moe & Izurieta (2004)
China	2 latrines	Plant ash mixed with faeces in ratio 1:3	pH: 9–10 temperature: −10 to 10 °C	**Controlled challenge test and organisms present in material:** After 3 months: >7 log reduction of *Salmonella typhimurium* phage 28B and faecal coliforms. 1% viability of *Ascaris*.	Wang (1999)[a]
China		No detailed information given	pH >8	**Controlled challenge test:** Inactivation of *Ascaris* within 120 days.	Lan et al. (2001)

[a] The other additives coal ash, sawdust and loess were also tested and resulted in lower pH and lower inactivation.

barrier, resulting in a higher safety level when the material is used as a fertilizer. High-temperature (thermophilic) composting of the dehydrated faeces may in some instances be considered as a secondary treatment, particularly if the contents of the toilet are to be used on food crops (Peasey, 2000).

Urine diversion systems

Urine is the most nutrient-rich fraction of the excreta (chapter 1). The aim of urine diversion is to collect urine for use as a fertilizer and to eliminate the eutrophicating discharge of nutrients into surface waters. Urine diversion may be practised using both composting and dehydration toilets. This practice enhances the drying or composting process by keeping out liquids. The collected urine can then be used as fertilizer after an appropriate storage period (chapter 4).

In urine diversion toilets, urine and faeces are collected separately. Low-, medium- and high-cost alternatives of this technology have been developed. The toilets come in both slab and sitting/pedestal toilet versions, and versions also exist for anal cleansing with water. Inserts for urine collection (Figure 5.5d) can be made from local material, but are also commercially available. In recent years, toilets made especially for urine diversion are available and used on all continents. In commercially produced urine-diverting toilets, the bowl/slab is divided into two compartments: a front one collecting urine and a rear one collecting faecal material (Figure 5.5a–c).

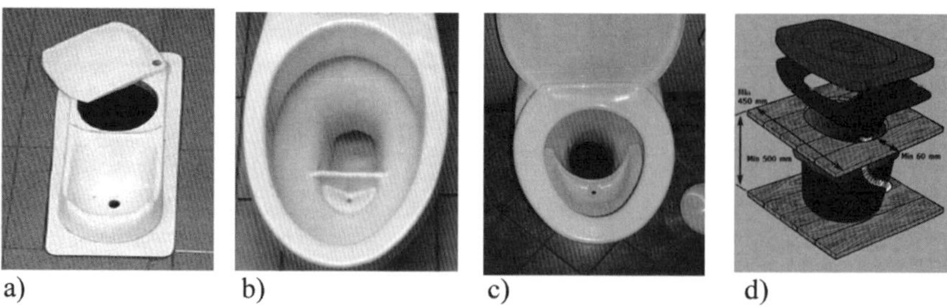

Figure 5.5

Examples of urine-diverting toilets: a) slab toilet, Guanxi province, China; b) double-flush urine diversion toilet; c) single-flush urine diversion toilet, Sweden; d) urine-diverting insert for a bucket toilet.

Urine diversion toilets with flushing apply either a single flush for urine with <0.5 litres or a double flush for either the urine or faecal matter with <4 litres. The single-flush system requires a straight chute down to the faecal collection chamber (Figure 5.6). The faecal matter is normally composted on site and the urine collected for use in agriculture (Winblad & Simpson-Hébert, 2004). Within pedestal toilets, a pan generally located towards the front of the defecating area collects the urine. Additional urinals can be used to collect urine from male users. If urinals are used, it is important to select models that use little water. In recent years, several new waterless urinals have appeared on the market. They have been tested in airports, hotels and universities and found to be without odour problems if properly maintained.

In the dual-flush system (Figure 5.7), the faecal matter is flushed into a sewer system and the urine collected separately. Dual-flush systems can be fitted in both new and existing urban areas with multistorey buildings (e.g. with a gravity urine collection system).

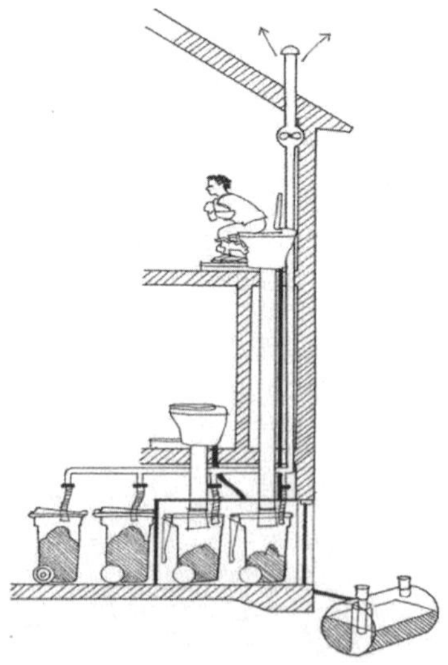

Figure 5.6

Technical layout of a single-flush urine diversion system in a two-storey apartment house (from Winblad & Simpson-Hébert, 2004)

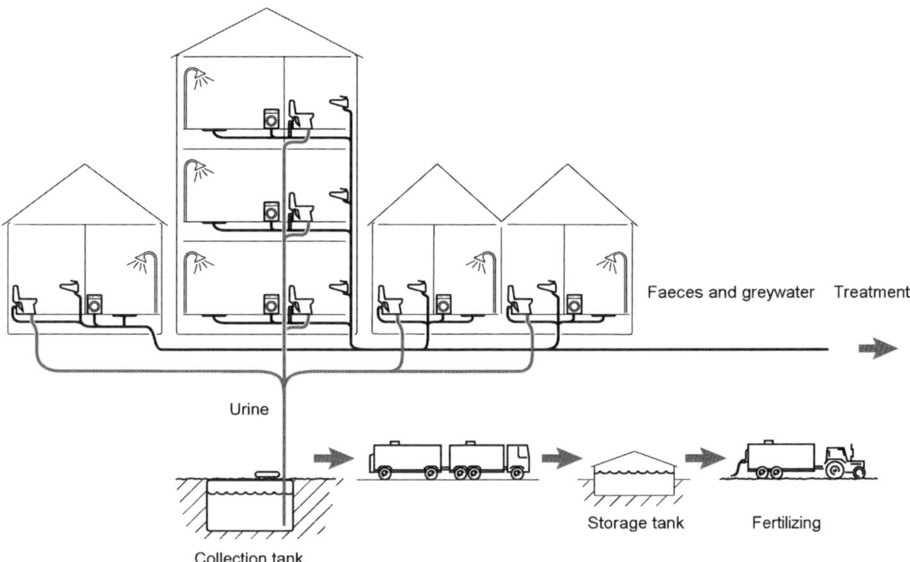

Figure 5.7
Layout for a dual-flush urine-diverting system. The urine is collected for use in agriculture, and the faecal matter is flushed away together with the greywater (Jönsson et al., 2000).

When the urine is collected using a urine diversion toilet, some faecal contamination may occur, which may pose a potential risk when using the urine. The cross-contaminating amounts are normally less than those for wastewater diluted 100-fold. Storage of the urine has been shown to give sufficient treatment with respect to pathogen reduction (Höglund, 2001). The sanitization is attributed to a rapid conversion of urea to ammonia, which increases the pH. The ammonia content together with the increase in pH have a sanitizing effect. Bacteria concentrations diminish quite quickly during storage, but prolonged storage is necessary in order to adequately reduce the number of viruses and protozoa (chapter 4).

Vacuum and low-flush gravity toilets

Vacuum and low-flush gravity toilets are used to collect blackwater (urine and faeces together) as concentrated as possible for further treatment, processing and use in agriculture. Vacuum toilets use 0.5–1.5 litres per flush; gravity toilets using as little as 1 litre per flush also exist. Blackwater collected using 1 litre per flush toilets has a low dry matter content (Jenssen, 2001). To treat the blackwater aerobically or anaerobically (section 5.2.3), additional organic matter (e.g. ground organic household waste) must be added (Figure 5.8).

The use of vacuum toilets provides a similar level of comfort as traditional flush toilets, but is potentially more hygienic due to air sucked into the toilet when flushing, thereby avoiding aerosols. The system is completely closed; should a leak occur, the negative pressure in the pipes reduces the risk of raw sewage spill. Vacuum toilet systems can be installed in multistorey buildings in urban situations.

The collected blackwater must be sanitized prior to agricultural use. This can be achieved using aerobic or anaerobic (yielding biogas) processes. Some vacuum toilets are available with urine diversion.

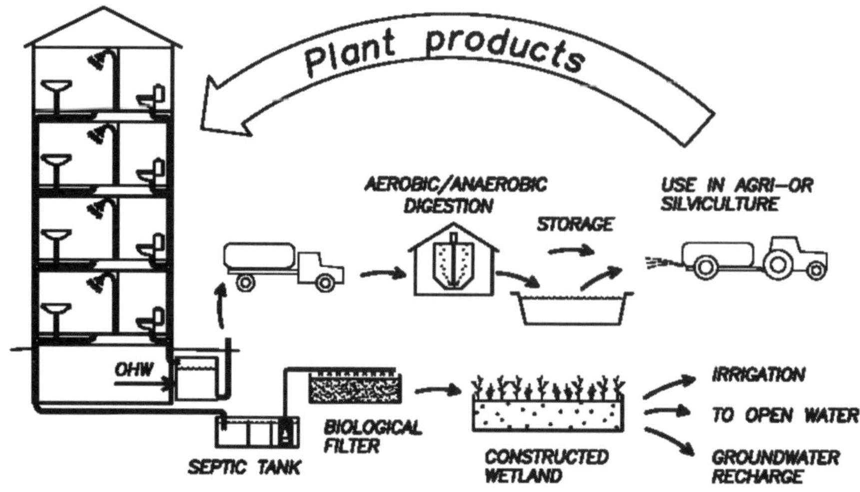

Figure 5.8
Example of a fully recycling system using vacuum or low-flush gravity toilets for separate collection of blackwater and separate treatment of greywater. Other greywater treatment options are given in section 5.2.4 (Jenssen, 2001).

Septic tank systems
Septic tank systems comprise all sanitation systems using a septic tank as the primary treatment step. In many developed countries, septic tanks followed by soil infiltration (leachfield or drainfield) constitute the major sanitation solution in rural areas. These systems normally treat combined wastewater (greywater and excreta). The pathogen removal in septic tanks is poor, and bacteria and viruses remain present in both the liquid and the solid phases The removal of helminth eggs can be expected to be <0.5 log, but suspended solids removal can potentially be used to assess the efficiency. The septic tank is the most common unit for on-site pretreatment of combined wastewater (greywater and excreta) and greywater. For the design of septic tanks, the reader is referred to Crites & Tchobanoglous (1998) or local plumbing codes.

Many of the inconveniences of conventional gravity sewers can be overcome through the use of small-diameter sewers transporting effluent from septic tanks, termed septic tank effluent gravity systems. Properly functioning septic tanks ensure that the solids settle and that the sewage network transports the liquid portion only. A planned programme for emptying the septic tanks is essential to successfully operate a small-diameter gravity sewer system. This is due to particles entering the system when the solid storage capacity of the septic tanks is reached. Provision of manholes is also essential throughout the network for maintenance and emergency interventions. Small-diameter gravity sewers are traditionally used for combined greywater and blackwater, but the same function is obtained using greywater septic tank effluent.

5.2.2 Handling and transport of excreta and sludge
Faeces and sludge need to be handled at various steps of the sanitation, treatment and use system. Handling and transport of faeces and sludge constitute critical points in a sanitation system from a health perspective, as people handling these materials may be exposed directly to pathogens, and there is a risk for accidental spill or intentional

dumping. The nature of materials that need to be handled varies, depending on their origin:

- dry materials from dehydration toilets or composting toilets, dried sludge and compost;
- sludge from septic and settling tanks, filters and anaerobic digesters, generally of liquid or semi-liquid consistency;
- contents from pit latrines with a consistency ranging from solid to liquid, often also containing solid waste.

Different options are available for the handling and transport of faeces and sludge:

- manual handling through excavation or emptying using buckets, transport in buckets or simple carts;
- mechanical emptying and transport, by vacuum tankers or trucks;
- pumping and piped transport of liquid sludge.

Piped sludge transport is the safest, but it is an option only if transport distance is limited and pumps can be afforded and managed.

The classical technology for emptying of septic tanks, pits and other excreta collections is by suction with a vacuum pump. A hose is introduced in the tank or pit, and the contents are sucked out. Sludge removal by suction pumps significantly reduces the direct contact of the workers with the sludge and is therefore the next safest technique available. The pump is usually connected to a truck-mounted tank of variable capacity. In this way, the truck can access the plot, empty the facility and then directly transport the sludge to the disposal or treatment site. Tanks may be mounted on carts pulled by a tractor or animals. Smaller units or vacuum tugs, consisting of smaller tanks and motor- or hand-driven vacuum pumps, may be used in situations where very narrow access does not allow large vehicles.

For blackwater tanks or urine tanks that contain no hard sludge or scum, a pipe with a quick coupling may be fitted to the holding tank, which reduces the time for emptying the tank and also reduces the potential for spills and possible human contact with untreated excreta (Jenssen et al., 2005).

From the human health risk perspective, a basic distinction should be made between sludges that, on collection, are still relatively fresh or contain a fair amount of recently deposited excreta (e.g. sludges from frequently emptied, unsewered public toilets) and sludges that have been retained in on-plot pits or vaults for months or years and are virtually free of pathogens. Blackwater constitutes high-risk material and exhibits characteristics similar to sludges collected at short intervals (e.g. from public toilets). Special care should therefore be taken against accidental contact and spill during emptying of latrine or toilet pits or vaults by vacuum trucks, where varying amounts of water or wastewater are collected alongside the accumulated solids. The content of helminth eggs may here be in the range of 500–6000 per litre (Koné & Strauss, 2004), which is higher than what can be expected in tropical sewage: 20–1000 per litre, according to Mara (1978).

Manual handling normally comprises the use of shovels and buckets and may demand that the workers have to step into the pit, thus exposing themselves to important health risks. Manual handling should be minimized if the material is not pretreated on site. However, manual handling will still be the final option when the use of vacuum pumps is excluded. Manual handling can be acceptable if the health risk to workers is minimized. Use of adequate protection measures by workers is absolutely necessary. Protection measures for handling of sludge include the use of protective clothing such as gloves and masks and good hygienic practices (hand washing after work, etc.). Workers must be aware of the nature of the health risks to which they are exposed, and they must know how to protect themselves. Training and targeted information are therefore the most powerful measures in addition to on-site treatment.

5.2.3 Treatment of blackwater and septic tank/faecal sludge

Low-cost treatment options

The faecal material collected from latrine or toilet pits may contain high numbers of pathogens if it has been stored for short periods of time (no more than 1–2 weeks) prior to collection. Secondary treatment serves to inactivate these pathogen levels below the tolerable risk threshold and the related guideline values. The solids fraction constitutes a valuable soil conditioner and fertilizer when stabilized and treated to the required hygienic quality. In contrast, the undiluted liquid fraction will, in most cases, not be usable in agriculture due to excessive salinity.

The solids–liquid separation processes, applicable for pumpable sludges, comprise settling and filtration and lead to a concentration of the pathogens trapped in the solids fraction. The sanitization process for this fraction will therefore be crucial, as the pathogen concentrations will have increased several-fold compared with the raw faecal sludge. Figure 5.9 schematically depicts an array of faecal sludge treatment processes and options, which may be suitable for low- or middle-income countries (Ingallinella et al., 2002).

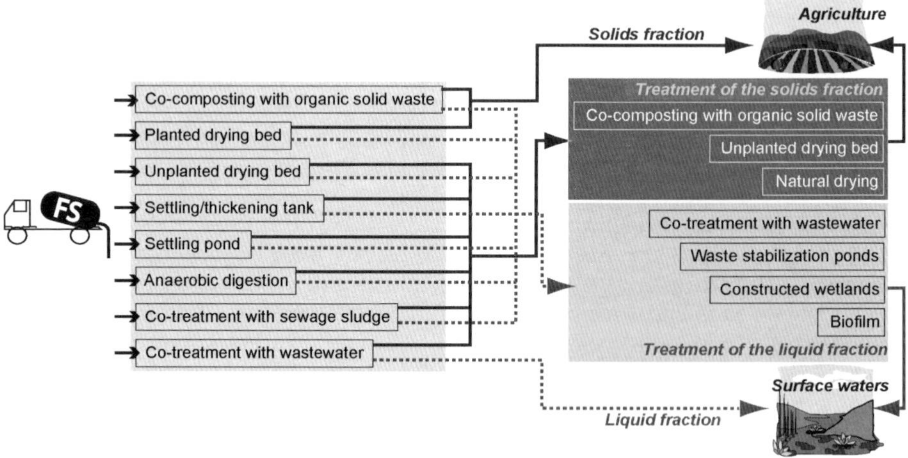

Figure 5.9

Low-cost options for treating faecal sludge (FS) and blackwater (Ingallinella et al., 2002)

Settling-thickening tanks or primary ponds can be used for solids–liquid separation. The former provide a liquid retention time of a few hours (enough to ensure quiescent settling of settleable solids), while the latter allow for several days or a few weeks of liquid retention and, hence, also allow for further sanitization and anaerobic degradation of organics. Batch-operated settling tanks can typically remove 60% of the suspended solids, while removal in settling ponds is >80% (Fernandez et al., 2004; Koné & Strauss, 2004). Helminth egg removals will be of the same order of magnitude.

Conventional sludge drying beds used for dewatering and drying of faecal sludge and anaerobic digester residue will reduce the faecal sludge volume applied by 50–80%. Sludge drying can reduce the water content to below 20–30%, which results in partial pathogen removal. The dried sludge still may contain pathogens, particularly helminth eggs, and should therefore receive further treatment (e.g. composting or prolonged storage) before use in agriculture. The drained liquid requires further treatment (e.g. in facultative ponds or in constructed wetlands) prior to discharge into a receiving water body.

Planted sludge drying or "humification" beds with a gravel/sand/soil filter planted with wetland plants such as, for example, reeds, bulrushes or cattails have the advantage over unplanted sludge drying beds, in that the roots of the plants create a porous structure in the accumulated solids, thus maintaining the dewatering capacity for several years in spite of an increased layer of accumulated sludge solids. Removal of accumulated biosolids is required at a much lower frequency, reducing contact. The extended storage of biosolids allows for biochemical stabilization and pathogen inactivation, resulting in a humus-like material, which is likely to require no or little additional storage to reach hygienic safety. Helminth egg viability in faecal sludge solids accumulated over three years in faecal sludge-fed planted drying beds was found to be less than 2% (Koottatep et al., 2004).

Waste stabilization pond systems comprise pretreatment units (tanks or ponds) for solids–liquid separation followed by a series of one or more anaerobic ponds and a facultative pond. Where faecal sludge is made up of substantial proportions (>30%) of sludges from unsewered public toilets, ammonia levels might be excessively high. In a tropical climate, the tolerable nitrogen level in the supernatant of primary settling units is 400 mg of NH_3-N + NH_4-N per litre (Heinss, Larmie & Strauss, 1998). Where waste stabilization ponds exist to treat municipal wastewater, faecal sludge is often mixed into the wastewater for co-treatment. This may create problems because the wastewater ponds were usually not designed to co-treat major loads of faecal sludge. To avoid problems, faecal sludge may be pretreated in primary settling-thickening ponds. Their effluent can then be co-treated with wastewater in facultative and maturation ponds. The faecal sludge settling ponds, which will also allow for anaerobic degradation of dissolved organics, enables the separation of the bulk of the solids and helminth eggs from the faecal sludge before reaching the main waste stabilization pond system.

Co-composting — i.e. the combined composting of faecal matter and organic solids waste — is practised all around the world, usually in small, informal and uncontrolled schemes or at a backyard scale. Most of this may proceed at ambient temperatures, with concomitant inefficient inactivation of pathogens. Thermophilic composting, however, can effectively sanitize and stabilize faecal sludge, faeces that have been pretreated in a urine diversion toilet or slurry from anaerobic treatment. If operating conditions required for thermophilic composting are adequate (moisture content 50–60%, carbon to nitrogen ratio 30–35 and mixing of bulking material to allow for sustained air passage), the temperature will rise to between 50 and 65 °C. Such temperatures will effectively inactivate pathogens. Fresh faecal sludge is normally too wet and exhibits too low a carbon to nitrogen ratio for optimal composting. Faecal sludge has to be dewatered prior to co-composting. Admixing of a relatively dry, carbon-rich bulking material such as organic municipal waste is required. The end-product of the aerobic composting process is an odourless, stabilized material with good properties as a soil conditioner and as a slow-release phosphorus fertilizer. Due to the complexity of the composting process, however, optimal thermophilic conditions throughout the composting mass can be guaranteed only if moisture content, bulking structure and carbon to nitrogen ratio are maintained and controlled throughout the thermophilic and maturation phases. Well operated thermophilic composting schemes can achieve close to 100% pathogen destruction, including very low helminth egg viabilities, if regular turnings are done during the 3- to 4-week thermophilic phase. Small-scale composting on a household level is less efficient and pathogen inactivation is incomplete, as the temperature increases only marginally above ambient. Prolonged storage would be the method of choice in that case. Composting is therefore best suited as a secondary off-site treatment.

Anaerobic digestion is a biological process that takes place in the absence of oxygen. The organic material is broken down, producing biogas (a mixture of methane, carbon dioxide and traces of other gases), water and remaining slurry. The slurry from the biogas reactor constitutes a valuable soil conditioner and fertilizer. This option is, in principle, suited to treat blackwater and higher-strength faecal sludge, which have not undergone substantial degradation. In India, in the order of 100 large-scale biogas plants are in operation, treating highly concentrated, fresh faecal sludge from public pour flush toilets. Small biogas digesters (Figure 5.10) serving one or a small number of households have become increasingly popular. The main goal of the household digesters is to produce biogas and provide the family with energy, mainly for cooking. The main input is animal manure from small household livestock, while human excreta and other organic wastes usually constitute the smaller fractions.

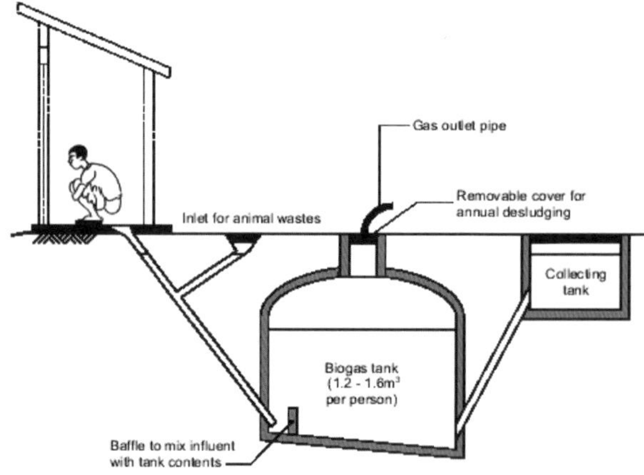

Figure 5.10
Household biogas digester for treatment of animal manure and human excreta

Pathogen reduction in mesophilic digestion is usually modest, with, on average, only 50% inactivation or 0.5 log cycles reduction of helminth egg viability (Feachem et al., 1983; Gantzer et al., 2001). Post-treatment, such as by sludge drying beds, thermophilic co-composting with organic bulking material or extended storage, is required to achieve the hygienic quality compatible with the guideline value.

High-cost treatment of faecal sludge and blackwater

In industrialized countries, treatment of faecal sludges or blackwater is largely based on established technologies. Frequently used options include extended aeration, anaerobic digestion, mechanically stirred sludge thickeners or chemical conditioning, followed by centrifuging or filter pressing. Complete pathogen removal can be achieved either in thermophilic processes or by processes especially designed for sanitization (e.g. pasteurization or high-alkaline treatment).

Large-scale biogas digesters are common for treating agricultural or organic municipal waste. Domestic wastewater or excreta from on-site sanitation systems or decentralized wastewater collection systems can also be co-treated in such digesters. Gas yields allow for the combined production of electricity and heat, and digester residues are used as fertilizers. Large digesters are usually heated and use mechanical agitation to maximize gas yields. The digestion process can be mesophilic or thermophilic. Thermophilic digestion yields higher gas production, allows for higher sludge loading rates and enables complete pathogen removal, but it requires more capital-extensive technology, higher energy inputs and higher operating skills. The residual liquid from thermophilic digesters can be safely used as a soil conditioner-cum-fertilizer, whereas slurries from mesophilic digesters have to be subjected to a separate sanitization process such as pasteurization, high-alkaline treatment, drying bed treatment or extended storage. Recent developments in biogas technology tend to combine anaerobic digestion with membrane filtration, allowing compact reactor volumes and complete pathogen removal. However, those technologies are still in the developmental stage.

Aerobic treatment of liquid organic waste is also termed liquid composting. It is based on slurry aeration, which induces a microbial degradation process by aerobic organisms, mainly bacteria. The process is exothermic, which means that the process generates heat. In a properly constructed and operated system, thermophilic temperatures are reached without additional heat sources, provided the relative organic content is sufficient The wastes are handled as liquids (dry matter content between 2% and 10%) and stabilized in the reactor at thermophilic temperatures between 55 and 60 °C with a hydraulic retention time of 5–7 days (Skjelhaugen, 1999). The process is run semicontinuously and is characterized by high oxygen utilization, low ammonia loss and no odour release (Skjelhaugen, 1999). Experimental investigations have shown that the pathogen removal is high and fulfils guideline targets (Norin et al., 1996).

Pathogen removal performance of treatment options and processes

Table 5.3 lists order of magnitude removals of helminth eggs for selected processes and low- and high-cost options for treating faecal sludges and blackwater. As expected, and by the nature of the processes involved — i.e. heat or high-alkaline treatment — high-cost options are more effective in helminth egg removal; that is, a greater log cycle reduction can be achieved in shorter retention time than with low-cost treatment options. This is a trade-off for higher investment and higher energy input.

5.2.4 Greywater

Greywater makes up the largest volume of the waste flow from households, with low nutrient and pathogen content. Simple treatment techniques such as soil infiltration; gravel filters, constructed wetlands or ponds may result in a level of pathogen reduction meeting the health-based targets. More complex methods, such as activated sludge, rotating biological contactors or membrane filtration, may also be used. The effluent, normally aimed for irrigation of agricultural crops in water-scarce regions, can also be used for groundwater recharge or industrial or urban reuse or discharged into surrounding watercourses (Werner et al., 2004).

Table 5.3 Helminth removal in different treatment processes for faecal sludge

Treatment option or process	Helminth egg log reduction	Duration	Reference
Low-cost			
Faecal sludge settling ponds	3	4 months	Fernandez et al. (2004)
Faecal sludge reed drying beds (constructed wetlands)	1.5	12 months	Koottatep et al. (2004)
Drying beds for dewatering (pretreatment)	0.5	0.3–0.6 months	Heinss, Larmie & Strauss (1998)
Composting (windrow thermophilic)	1.5–2.0	3 months	Koné et al. (2004)
pH elevation >9	3	6 months	Chien et al. (2001)
Anaerobic (mesophilic)	0.5	0.5–1.0 month	Feachem et al. (1983); Gantzer et al. (2001)
High-cost			
pH elevation >12	3		Gantzer et al. (2001)
Thermophilic, in-vessel (aerobic/anaerobic)	3	1–5 days	Haug (1993); Eller, Norin & Stenström (1996)

Source control and water conservation are part of the general management of greywater. This relates to the use of environmentally friendly household chemicals and reducing faecal input as well as reducing the amount of water to be treated. Progressive planning can calculate a mean amount of 80 litres of greywater per person per day (Ridderstolpe, 2004). In industrialized countries, excess amounts of detergents are responsible for substantial BOD input, and greywater will also contain excess amounts of grease and oil originating from food preparation. If greywater is to be used for irrigation, liquid soaps containing potassium are preferred, since hard soaps often contain sodium, which increases the risk of soil salinization. More information on greywater volume and composition has been given in chapter 1.

Greywater collection is normally based on a pipe system with smaller-diameter pipes than for combined wastewater and equipped with ventilation for air and odour evacuation and water traps. The final discharge or use of the water determines the extent of treatment needed. Before discharge to streams or use in irrigation or groundwater recharge, the treatment should safeguard the hygienic quality. For groundwater recharge, substantial reduction of BOD and suspended solids is normally needed to prevent clogging of the recharge basins or wells. For domestic reuse, more sophisticated tertiary treatment may be necessary

A range of treatment alternatives is available for on-site or small-scale decentralized greywater treatment (Figure 5.11). The most common options are briefly described below. These can also be used for treatment of combined wastewater, but have to be designed accordingly.

Pretreatment/solid–liquid separation

Pretreatment is always needed to avoid clogging of the subsequent treatment step. It consists of a solid–liquid separation that reduces the amounts of particles and fat in the effluent by septic tanks, settling tanks, ponds or filter systems such as filter bags.

The most common pretreatment unit for greywater as well as for treatment of combined wastewater (greywater and excreta) on site is a septic tank (see Septic tank systems in section 5.2.1). The pathogen removal in septic tanks is poor (normally <0.5 log) and depends on the efficiency of particle removal. A regular (yearly) inspection is recommended to prevent problems with particle overflow.

For small systems, such as a single dwelling, an alternative to the septic tank may be filter bags from natural or synthetic material that produce the same effluent quality. A homeowner can remove such bags with proper personal protection against exposure to the material, which may contain pathogens. The bags can be composted together with their content if they are made of natural fibre or dried and reused if they are made of synthetic fabrics.

Home-made screens or filters made of fine gravel, straw or branches may also be appropriate prior to soil infiltration in small-scale domestic systems in hot climates. In small systems, direct use of greywater is also possible (i.e. to a mulch bed where water is used for growing plants or trees).

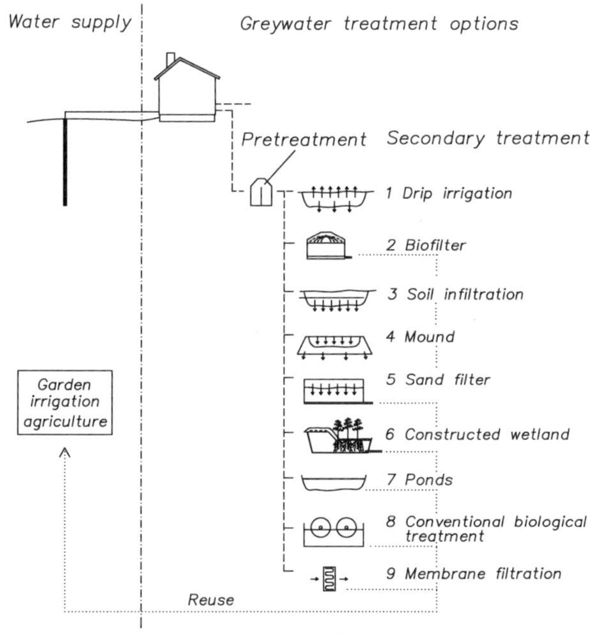

Figure 5.11
Greywater treatment options

Soil infiltration

Soil infiltration is a simple and suitable method for on-site greywater treatment, for which comprehensive experience exists regarding both separated greywater and combined wastewater. It is, for example, the primary system for on-site and decentralized wastewater treatment in the United States. The treatment efficiencies are high (normally >2 logs for both bacteria and viruses and >3 logs for parasitic protozoa), thus giving a similar reduction efficiency as a traditional wastewater treatment plant (Siegrist, Tyler & Jenssen, 2000).

After the pretreatment, the effluent is distributed to the soil through open ponds or shallow trenches or infiltration basins (Figure 5.12).

The water percolates down through an unsaturated zone to the groundwater (saturated zone). Most of the treatment occurs in the unsaturated zone. The size and

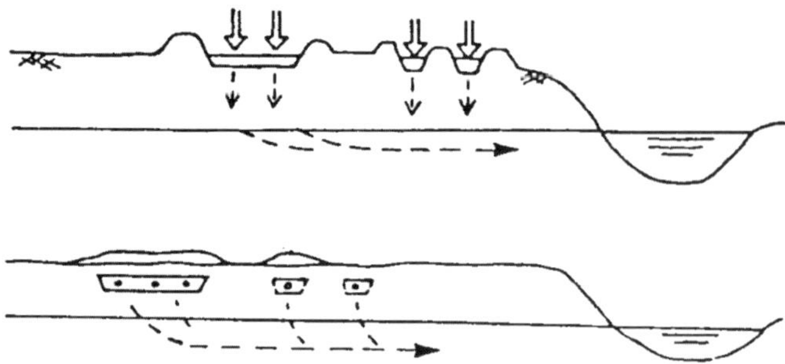

Figure 5.12
Infiltration in open basins/ponds (above) and in buried shallow trenches (below); the percolation down to the groundwater and subsequent flow towards a stream are indicated

load of the system need to account for the local soil conditions to keep the flow unsaturated, which assures optimum conditions for filtering of pathogens. Unsaturated flow also assures aerobic conditions that generally promote a more rapid die-off of pathogens.

Soil infiltration systems should not be used where the groundwater quality may be endangered. The necessary separation distance to groundwater varies depending on soil type and system design (Siegrist, Tyler & Jenssen, 2000). Virus and bacteria removal as well as phosphorus sorption are enhanced by soils rich in iron and aluminium oxides (brown- and red-coloured soils). Disposal systems should always be downslope and as far as possible from water wells to protect possible water supplies from contamination. Impermeable soils, shallow rock, shallow water tables or very permeable soils such as coarse sand or gravelly soils are normally considered unsuitable sites. For permeable soils, a layer of sand 30–50 cm in the bottom of the infiltration trench will enhance the retention capacity for microorganisms. Elevated systems (mounds) can also be designed to overcome limitations in the local soil conditions (USEPA, 2002). For information on siting and design, the reader is referred to Jenssen & Siegrist (1990, 1991), Siegrist, Tyler & Jenssen (2000) and USEPA (2002).

Drip irrigation

Drip irrigation is a shallow soil infiltration system where the plant uptake of water and nutrients is optimized, thus minimizing vertical percolation to the groundwater. The system may be simple or advanced, with pressurized distribution of the liquid. Localized irrigation is estimated to provide an additional pathogen reduction of 2–4 log units, depending on whether the harvested part of the crop is in contact with the soil (see Volume 2 of the Guidelines) (NRMMC & EPHCA, 2005).

Ponds

Wastewater stabilization ponds are developed for combined wastewater treatment but are also suitable for greywater. Waste stabilization pond treatment systems usually consist of a number of ponds linked in series and should be designed to minimize hydraulic short-circuiting. For greywater treatment, an anaerobic stage is usually not required. The design criteria for helminth egg and *E. coli* removal are discussed in Volume 2 of the Guidelines. A properly designed series of waste stabilization ponds can easily reduce faecal coliform numbers from 10^8 per 100 ml to $<10^3$ per 100 ml. In tropical environments (20–30 °C), well designed and properly operated waste stabilization ponds can achieve a 2–4 log unit removal of viruses, a 3–6 log unit removal of bacterial pathogens, a 1–2 log unit removal of protozoan (oo)cysts and a 3 log unit removal of helminth eggs; the precise values depend on the number of ponds in series and their retention times (Mara & Silva, 1986; Oragui et al., 1987; Grimason et al., 1993; Mara, 2004). The removal is mainly by sedimentation for protozoan (oo)cysts and helminth eggs, while viruses are removed by adsorption onto solids and bacteria by inactivation by several mechanisms, such as temperature, pH and light intensity (Curtis, Mara & Silva, 1992).

Effluent storage reservoirs can also be used for greywater treatment in arid and semi-arid countries. Due to the organic load, a pretreatment step may be needed. Effluent storage and reservoirs may, if properly designed, operated and maintained, result in pathogen removals within the same range as waste stabilization ponds.

Constructed wetlands

Artificial shallow ponds vegetated with macrophytes are normally referred to as constructed wetlands. A pond filled with a porous medium is referred to as a subsurface flow constructed wetland (Figure 5.13), where the porous medium can be sand, gravel, lightweight aggregate or other, suited to support the macrophytes and to have a sufficient hydraulic conductivity to transport water horizontally through the root zone. Fine-grained soils as silt or clays are not suitable, due to their low hydraulic conductivity and consequently high risk for surfacing of flow and short-circuiting of the system, resulting in poor treatment performance.

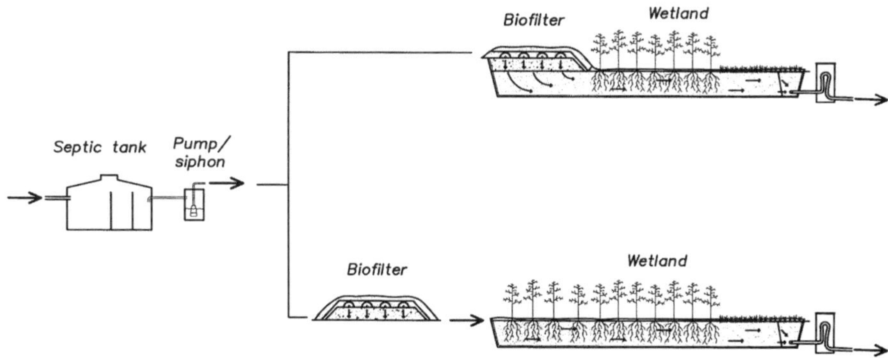

Figure 5.13

A subsurface flow wetland with and without integrated biofilter (Source: post-graduate training materials prepared by P. Jenssen & A. Heistad, Agricultural University of Norway, Aas, Norway, 2000)

The geometry of a subsurface flow constructed wetland is based on hydraulic calculations. In a cold climate where the plants are seasonally dormant, aerobic pretreatment is recommended (Jenssen et al., 2005) to achieve high removal of BOD and nitrogen during the cold period, and deeper systems are used to allow for the upper part to freeze while the water still flows lower down. In a cold-temperate climate, 1-m-deep systems are recommended, while in a warm climate, 0.4–0.6 m depths are the most common.

Constructed wetlands with subsurface flow are well suited for greywater treatment. Constructed wetlands give a high reduction of BOD and total nitrogen, while phosphorus removal is dependent on the adsorption capacity of the media (Zhu,

1998). Constructed wetlands can reduce the pathogen load significantly and can produce an effluent with <1000 thermotolerant coliforms per 100 ml (Jenssen & Vråle, 2004; Jenssen et al., 2005). Normally, the reduction of pathogens (as well as of somatic coliphages) depends on the type and size of the porous media and the retention time. The macrophytes may also enhance the removal (Franceys, Pickford & Reed, 1992). When using iron-rich sand and allowing a residence time of more than one week, a removal of 3 logs of indicator bacteria and a substantial virus removal have been achieved.

In warm climates where plants do not have a long dormant period, a greywater treatment wetland can be constructed without a pretreatment biofilter, and the dosing system (pump/siphon) can also be omitted. However, with a biofilter, more compact systems can be made (Jenssen & Vråle, 2004) for urban applications.

Sand filters/vertical-flow constructed wetlands

The sand filter is a well proven method for wastewater purification, which, over the last two decades, has been used with plants (often termed vertical-flow wetland) and is well suited for greywater treatment. The water flow is a vertical unsaturated flow (as in unplanted sand filters), and the treatment equal to the unsaturated zone in a soil infiltration system. The purification performance is, as for soil infiltration systems, dependent on the hydraulic loading and the sand texture and surface chemistry of the sand grains. Typical loadings are in the range of 2–10 cm/day. In fine- and medium-grain sands, more than a 3 log reduction of indicator bacteria can be expected, the BOD removal is >80% and effluent suspended solids is <5 mg/l (Jenssen & Siegrist, 1990). Bacteria, virus and phosphorus removal is enhanced when using sand rich in iron or aluminium oxides. Aeration is improved and short-circuiting avoided if the filter is constructed with sloping sand walls on the sides of the gravel or distribution layer (Figure 5.14).

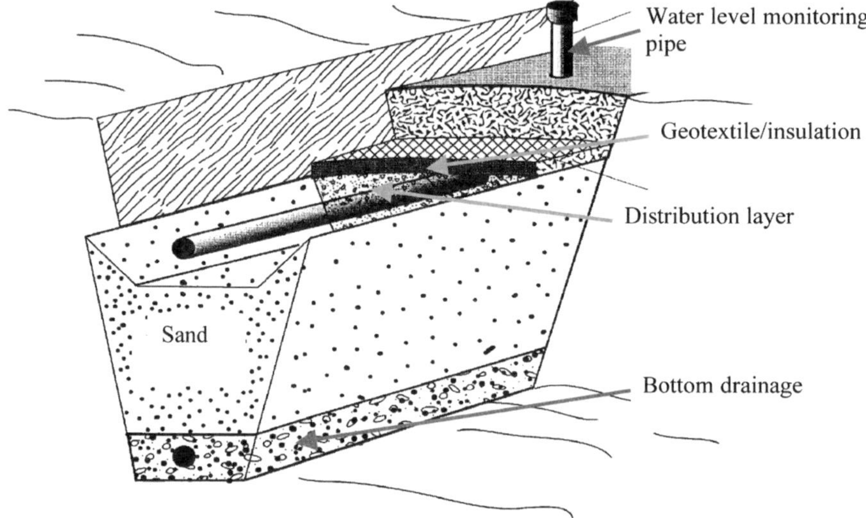

Figure 5.14
Sand filter design with sloping sand walls at the level of the distribution pipe

Biofilters

Single-pass vertical-flow biofilters as pretreatment to constructed wetlands use lightweight aggregates of 2–10 mm grain size, but other media can act as support for the biofilm with maintained performance for BOD reduction (Jenssen et al., 2005). In Malaysia, crushed coconut shell is suggested as a biofilter medium. High removals of indicator bacteria have been observed during intermittent filtration, with hydraulic loading rate, media grain size and retention time being the most important factors (Stevik et al., 1998, 1999). Pretreatment in a biofilter aerates the greywater and reduces BOD and bacteria, so higher loading rates can be obtained for the subsequent wetland or infiltration system (Heistad, Jenssen & Frydenlund, 2001). For greywater loading rates up to 110 cm/day, a >70% removal of BOD and ~5 log reduction of indicator bacteria have been achieved (Jenssen & Vråle, 2004). A uniform distribution of the water over the filter surface can be obtained using siphons, tipping buckets or a pump and a spray nozzle.

Mulch beds and greywater gardens

Dishpan dump, drain mulch basins and similar simple applications of direct use of greywater do not need pretreatment. The mulch bed may be constructed beside trees or berry bushes and the bed excavated and filled with gravel, bark or wood chips. The application and design aim to ensure that water is spread evenly over the area, based on the plant needs. Normally, water is applied by gravity, but a pressurized system can also be used.

Greywater gardens are a similar technology, where greywater is treated in a planted constructed wetland. Contrary to mulch beds, which need to be replaced when the organic material is decomposed, greywater gardens are permanent installations. Pretreatment is recommended to avoid clogging, and subsurface application minimizes the exposure of workers in the gardens.

Activated sludge

Activated sludge systems have not been extensively used for greywater treatment. It is assumed that the treatment efficiency will be low if greywater is low in biodegradable carbon, which was shown by Gunther (2000). Activated sludge systems must generally be succeeded by additional treatment to achieve more than a 3 log reduction of faecal indicators.

Rotating biological contactors

In Germany, a successful system using rotating biological contactors has been developed. The system is compact and can be located, for example, in the basement of an apartment building. In order to achieve a reduction of faecal indicators above 3 logs, the system is equipped with ultraviolet disinfection.

Membrane filtration

Membrane processes use a semipermeable membrane and osmotic or lower pressure differential to force water through the membrane as permeate, with dissolved solids or other constituents captured as retentate. Membranes are often made of organic polymers, but new types of inorganic polymers as well as ceramic and metallic membranes are under development. The basic membrane systems include microfiltration, ultrafiltration, nanofiltration and reverse osmosis, each of which retains a different range of particle sizes. Problems with operation and maintenance with membrane treatment may occur through fouling as a result of material buildup, blocking fluid flow across the membrane. Reverse osmosis is particularly susceptible to blockage and therefore requires pretreatment. However, membrane filtration offers a >6 log removal of microorganisms and may be applied for upgrading of treated greywater to meet requirements for in-house use.

6 MONITORING AND SYSTEM ASSESSMENT

Monitoring has three different purposes: validation, or proving that the system is capable of meeting its design requirements; operational monitoring, which provides information regarding the functioning of individual system components related to health protection measures; and verification, which usually takes place at the end of the process (e.g. treated excreta and greywater, crop contamination) to ensure that the system is achieving its specified targets.

The most effective means of consistently ensuring safety in source separating systems and the final use of the end-products in agriculture is through the use of a comprehensive risk assessment and risk management approach that encompasses all steps in the process, from the generation and use of excreta and greywater to the consumption of the agricultural product. This approach is captured in the Stockholm Framework (see chapter 2). Three components are important: system assessment; identifying control measures and methods for monitoring them; and developing a management plan. System assessment and its components are discussed in section 6.2.

The combination of health protection measures adopted in a particular excreta and greywater use scheme requires regular monitoring to ensure that the system continues to function effectively. Monitoring, in the sense of observing, inspecting and verifying, is not sufficient on its own. Institutional arrangements must be established for the information collected in this way to provide feedback to those who implement the health protection measures. The structure of the monitoring system is site specific and may vary in size and function, but its planning and operation will be concentrated around simple questions, such as:

1) What information should be collected?
2) How often and by whom should this information be collected?
3) To whom will this monitoring information be given?
4) What decisions will be taken on the basis of the monitoring information?
5) How can those decisions be implemented?

This requires operational guidelines and verification procedures with which the monitoring results can be compared. Decisions can be implemented either on the user or community level or by an implementing or operating agency for corrective actions or enforcement. In the case of surveillance by an enforcement agency (e.g. a Ministry of Health), the agency has legal powers to enforce compliance with quality standards and other legislation.

6.1 Monitoring functions

The three functions of monitoring are each used for different purposes at different times, as briefly summarized in Table 6.1. Validation is performed at the beginning when a new system is developed or when new processes are added. It is used to test or prove that the system is capable of meeting the specified targets. Operational monitoring is used on a routine basis to indicate that the system is working as expected. Monitoring of this type relies on simple measurements (e.g. use, storage time, functionality) that can be read quickly so that decisions can be made in time to remedy a potential problem. Verification is used to show that the end-product (e.g. excreta, crop contamination) meets microbial quality specifications. Information from verification monitoring is mainly relevant in large collection systems and should not be applied at a household level. When collected periodically from larger systems, verification monitoring information will usually not prevent a hazard break-through, but can indicate trends over time (e.g. whether the efficiency of a specific process or system is increasing or decreasing).

Table 6.1 Definitions of monitoring functions

Function	Definition
Validation	Testing the system and its individual components to obtain evidence that they are capable of meeting the specified targets (i.e. microbial reduction targets). Should take place when a new system is developed or the treatment is changed.
Operational monitoring	The act of conducting a planned sequence of observations or measurements of control parameters to assess whether a control measure is operating within design specifications. Emphasis is given to parameters that can be measured quickly and easily and that can indicate if the system is functioning properly. Operational monitoring data should help managers to make corrections that can prevent hazard break-through.
Verification	The application of methods, procedures, tests and other evaluations, in addition to those used in operational monitoring, to determine compliance with the system design parameters and/or whether the system meets specified requirements (e.g. microbial testing for *E. coli* or helminth eggs).

Source: Adapted from NRMMC & EPHCA (2005).

6.2 System assessment

The first step in developing a risk management system is to form a multidisciplinary team of professionals with a thorough understanding of different aspects of the system for recirculation of excreta or greywater as resources. Typically, such a team would include agriculture experts, engineers, environmental health specialists and public health authorities. In most settings, the team would include members from several institutions, and there should be some independent members, such as from universities.

Effective management of the excreta/greywater system requires a comprehensive understanding of the range and magnitude of hazards that may be present, what determines the associated risk levels and the ability of existing processes, barriers and infrastructure to manage actual or potential risks. It also requires an assessment of capabilities to meet targets. When a new system or an upgrade of an existing system is being planned, the first step in developing a risk management plan is the collection and evaluation of all available relevant information and consideration of what risks may arise during the entire process. Figure 6.1 illustrates the consecutive steps in the development of a risk management plan.

The assessment and evaluation of an excreta/greywater system could be enhanced through a flow diagram. Such diagrams provide an overview description of the system, including the identification of sources of hazards and health protection measures. To ensure accuracy, flow diagrams should be validated by visually checking them against features observed on the ground. Identification of the potential occurrence of hazards in the system combined with information concerning the effectiveness of existing controls form a base for an assessment of whether health-based targets can be achieved with the existing health protection measures or improvements thereof. All elements of the system should be considered concurrently, as well as the interactions and influences between elements and their overall effect.

6.3 Validation

Validation is concerned with obtaining system evidence on the performance of control measures, both individually and collectively. It should ensure the system's capability

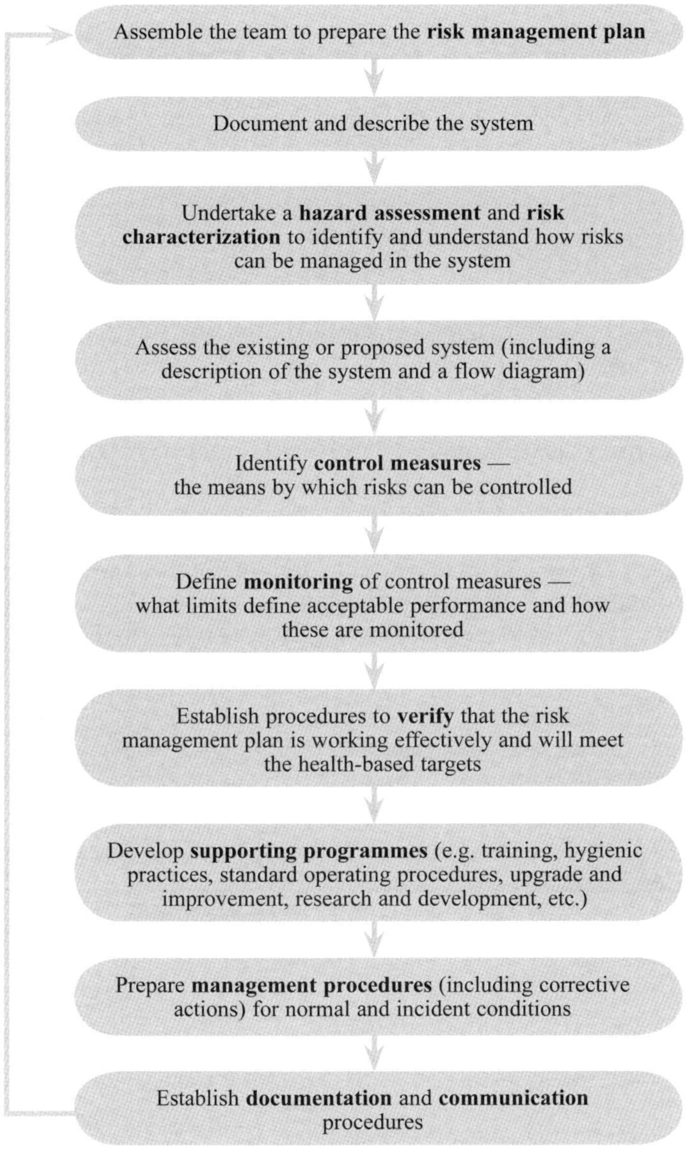

Assemble the team to prepare the **risk management plan**

Document and describe the system

Undertake a **hazard assessment** and **risk characterization** to identify and understand how risks can be managed in the system

Assess the existing or proposed system (including a description of the system and a flow diagram)

Identify **control measures** — the means by which risks can be controlled

Define **monitoring** of control measures — what limits define acceptable performance and how these are monitored

Establish procedures to **verify** that the risk management plan is working effectively and will meet the health-based targets

Develop **supporting programmes** (e.g. training, hygienic practices, standard operating procedures, upgrade and improvement, research and development, etc.)

Prepare **management procedures** (including corrective actions) for normal and incident conditions

Establish **documentation** and **communication** procedures

Figure 6.1
Development of a risk management plan (WHO, 2004a)

of meeting specified microbial reduction targets and design criteria. Validation is used to test or prove design criteria. It should be conducted before a new risk management process is put into place (e.g. for greywater and excreta treatment, application and crop harvest), when system components are upgraded (e.g. new toilet collection design) or when procedures are added (e.g. composting or pH elevation of excreta; irrigation regimes of greywater). It can also be used to test different combinations of processes to maximize process efficiency. Validation of an on-site excreta treatment/storage system could provide data on die-off of different enteric pathogens under existing treatment conditions (e.g. temperature, moisture content, after addition of lime, etc.).

Validation can be conducted at the facility scale or on a test scale, starting with consideration of existing data on site, data from other facilities, the scientific literature, regulation and legislation departments and professional bodies, historical data and supplier knowledge. These data may be compared or supplemented with laboratory or pilot-level evaluations of the components and overall system under the prevailing conditions taking into account seasonal variations. Validation is not intended for day-to-day management; thus, parameters that may be inappropriate for operational monitoring can be used (WHO, 2004a).

6.4 Operational monitoring

Control measures are actions implemented in the system that prevent, reduce or eliminate contamination and are identified in system assessment. They include, for example, on-site excreta treatment/storage facilities, use of personal protection during emptying, waste application techniques and adequate time between application and harvest. If collectively operating properly, they would ensure that health-based targets are met.

Operational monitoring is the execution of planned observations or measurements to assess whether the control measures in an excreta and greywater use system are operating properly. It is possible to set limits for control measures (e.g. minimum storage time, temperature and conditions during composting, etc.), monitor those limits and take corrective action in response to a detected deviation before the contamination passes through the system. Operational monitoring should take place around system parameters that indicate the potential for increased risk of hazard break-through. It is facilitated by simple measurements that can be taken quickly. These types of controls can easily be performed within a community, by village committees, community workers, etc. Examples of parameters that can be monitored are presented in Table 6.2.

Table 6.2 Validation, operational and verification monitoring parameters for different control measures

Control measures (numbers refer to control points in Figure 6.2)	Validation requirements	Operational monitoring parameters and technical measures	Verification monitoring
Excreta and greywater treatment	Effectiveness of treatment processes at inactivating/removing pathogens and indicator organisms (*E. coli*, trematode eggs, other helminths, e.g. *Ascaris*)	Parameters ensuring sufficient treatment, design, limiting vector transmission and secondary transmission and reducing personal contact	For faeces and greywater: *E. coli* Helminth eggs (*Ascaris*) For urine: Faecal cross-contamination
I. Toilet	Reduction efficiency against enteric bacteria, viruses and parasites	Design that facilitates cleaning, elevated and/or lined collection chamber (no seepage to groundwater or environment), fly control measures (tight-fitting lid, ventilation pipe with screen) Clean water and soap for hand washing available	Ensure appropriate construction and use

Table 6.2 (continued)

Control measures (numbers refer to control points in Figure 6.2)	Validation requirements	Operational monitoring parameters and technical measures	Verification monitoring
II. Primary handling – collection and transport	Reduced direct contact with insufficiently treated material	Adequate storage time in double-vault toilets Ash, lime or other means of reducing microorganisms at toilet Collecting and transporting mechanisms that reduce contact, e.g. removal containers Gloves, washing hands, personal protection	Ensure adequate handling and adequate treatment
III. Treatment	Reduced direct contact with insufficiently treated material and environmental contamination	Suitable choice of location; treatment in closed systems; information signs in place Wearing gloves and protective clothing; washing hands; avoiding contact in treatment areas	Ensure adequate handling and adequate treatment
Health and hygiene promotion	Testing of promotional materials with relevant stakeholder groups	Local programmes in operation Promotional materials available Promotion included in school curriculum	Increased awareness of health and hygiene issues in key stakeholder groups Improved practices
IV. Secondary handling – use, fertilizing	Reduced direct contact with insufficiently treated material and environmental contamination	Wearing gloves Washing hands Equipment used	Informed farmers using excreta Special equipment available
V. Fertilized field	The amount of time needed for pathogen die-off under different climatic conditions and for different pathogens/ indicators between waste application and crop harvest to ensure minimal contamination	Working excreta into the ground Information and signs Avoiding overfertilization	Analyse plant contamination
VI. Fertilized crop –produce restriction	Survey of product consumers to identify species always eaten after thorough cooking Analysis of marketability of different species/crops Economic viability of growing products not for human consumption Harvesting, transport and trade Consumption Contamination of hands, kitchen utensils, food	Harvesting and transport practices Withholding time between fertilization and harvest Types of crops grown in excreta use areas Crops cooked before eating	Testing of excreta/greywater to ensure that it meets WHO microbial reduction targets Proper preparation and cooking of food products Domestic and food hygiene Hand washing

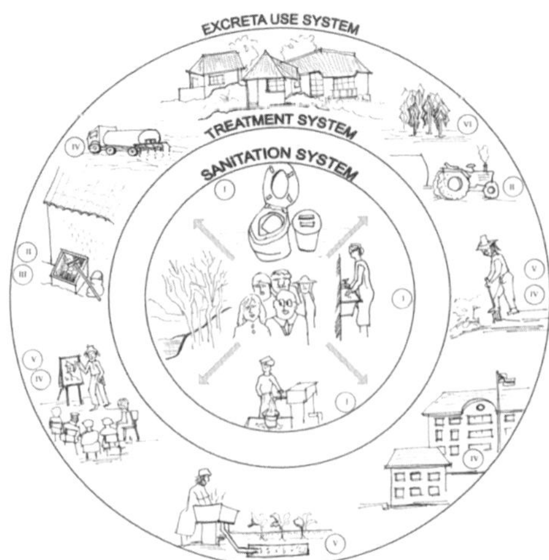

Figure 6.2
Elements of an excreta monitoring system

The frequency of operational monitoring varies with the nature of the control measure. If monitoring shows that a limit does not meet specifications, then there is the potential for a hazard break-through. For the treatment of excreta, storage time and temperature can be monitored to indicate pathogen inactivation. The emptying process, either for on-site units or for faecal sludge, the transportation system as well as the withholding time on the fields are other examples of simple monitoring. For a greywater system, the faecal cross-contamination and following adequate treatment are central. Open greywater systems should be controlled for mosquito breeding. For faecal sludge, the indiscriminate dumping of chemicals may warrant control. In most cases, operational monitoring will be based on simple and rapid observations or tests rather than complex microbial or chemical tests. Instead, these may be a part of validation and verification activities rather than of operational monitoring. Monitoring needs to be conducted in such a way that it provides statistically meaningful information (e.g. sample duplicates), is directed at controlling the most important hazards and can inform changes to health protection measures. A monitoring programme should be designed in such a way that it can be performed within the technical and financial resources of any given situation. The objective is timely monitoring of control measures with a logically based sampling plan, to minimize negative public health impacts (WHO, 2004a).

6.5 Verification

Verification is the use of methods, procedures or tests in addition to those used in operational monitoring to determine if the performance of the greywater/excreta use system is in compliance with the stated objectives outlined by the health-based targets and/or whether the system needs modification and revalidation.

For microbial reduction targets, verification is likely to include microbial analysis. This relates mainly to the faecal/faecal sludge fraction and greywater in source separating systems, but not directly to the urine fraction, since the latter usually results in a too rapid die-off of *E. coli* to serve its monitoring purpose. The other fractions involve the analysis of faecal indicator microorganisms; in some circumstances, verification may also include assessment of specific pathogen densities (e.g. helminth ova). Verification of the microbial quality may be undertaken by local public health agencies. Approaches to verification include testing either after treatment or at the point of application or use. Verification of the microbial quality of the wastes often includes testing for *E. coli*. While *E. coli* is a useful indicator, this organism has limitations, and its absence will not necessarily indicate the absence of other pathogens. Under certain circumstances, it may be desirable to include more resistant microorganisms, such as *Ascaris* or bacteriophages (viruses that infect bacteria), as indicators for other microbial groups and relate this to a microbial risk assessment of the system.

6.6 Small systems

Validation, operational monitoring and verification are important steps to identify and eventually mitigate public health issues that might be associated with use of excreta and greywater in agriculture. However, in some situations, such use can be difficult to monitor, because it takes place mostly at the subsistence level with small facilities spread out in many locations or is practised indirectly and informally (e.g. in urban areas or in small-scale operations). Additionally, and in comparison, open defecation frequently occurs, and much of the wastewater use in agriculture that is practised is indirect and informal (e.g. irrigation with faecally contaminated surface waters). Countries and local authorities may have limited budgets for validation and monitoring and thus will need to develop validation and monitoring programmes based upon the most important local public health issues, the availability of professional staff and access to laboratory facilities.

With many household-level units, the national health or food safety authority may choose to validate health protection measures at a central research site and then disseminate information to relevant stakeholders, e.g. through the development of locally adopted guidelines, public health outreach workers, community committees, health associations or local stakeholder workshops. For small systems, operational monitoring should focus on visual inspections and safety audits without requiring difficult or expensive laboratory testing.

Verification monitoring may be easier to conduct. Data from public health surveillance for faecal–oral diseases, schistosomiasis, intestinal helminth infections and other locally important diseases should be used to adjust health protection measures as necessary.

6.7 Other types of monitoring

Periodically, the microbial contamination of fertilized crops should be tested. Products should be tested for *E. coli* and helminth eggs where they are a hazard.

Direct measurement of specific health outcomes (e.g. diarrhoeal disease, intestinal helminth infections, schistosomiasis and vector-borne diseases) is possible and can be assessed periodically in exposed populations. This has been discussed in the context of the Stockholm Framework in chapter 2.

7
SOCIOCULTURAL ASPECTS

Human behaviour is a key determinant of the transmission of excreta-related diseases. The feasibility of changing certain behavioural patterns in order to optimize safety in the introduction of excreta or wastewater use schemes or to reduce disease transmission in existing schemes can be assessed only with a prior understanding of the cultural values attached to the social preferences that determine behaviour and practices. Cultural beliefs vary so widely in different parts of the world that it is not possible to assume that any of the practices that have evolved in relation to excreta and wastewater use in one place can be readily transferred elsewhere; a thorough assessment of the local sociocultural context is always necessary. There appears to have been a positive correlation, however, between the phenomenon of traditional "waste" use in societies and their population density. This is referred to as the "nutritional imperative." Societies that use excreta or have used it in the recent past in agriculture or aquaculture are the most densely populated: Europe, India, China and South-east Asia (Edwards, 1992).

Culture varies, and social groups have their own norms and practices with respect to excretion, which will vary with age, gender, education, class, religion, marital status, employment and physical capacity (Tanner, 1995). Social change may put attitudes and norms under pressure, depending on what is considered modern or fashionable or what customs can be retained in new environments (Drangert, 2004b). They may also evolve as technology advances and governance structures and procedures are updated. Sociocultural aspects of excreta and greywater use in agriculture are outlined in the sections below.

7.1 Perceptions of excreta and greywater use

Human society has developed different sociocultural responses to the use of untreated excreta, ranging from abhorrence through disaffection and indifference to predilection. Most religions provide recommendations on how to manage excreta and have shaped people's perceptions. Also, cultural, physical and social aspects condition the views of use.

In Africa, the Americas and Europe, use of fresh excreta is generally regarded with disaffection. However, conditioning makes caretakers perceive faeces of children and elderly as inoffensive, and the same applies to one's own faeces. Products fertilized with raw excreta are regarded as tainted or defiled, but large agricultural areas in many countries are fertilized with raw sewage, and the products find consumers (see Volume 2 of the Guidelines). Negative views are less articulated in relation to excreta-derived compost or wastewater sludge commonly used in agriculture, horticulture and land reclamation schemes.

In contrast, fresh human excreta have been used in agriculture and aquaculture in Asian countries for thousands of years. This practice is in social accord with the Japanese and Chinese traditions of frugality and reflects an economic appreciation of soil fertility. This has evolved in response to the need to feed large populations with limited land availability, which makes it a necessity to use all fertilizing resources available. However, access to cheap chemical fertilizers has changed the practices in Japan (Ishikawa, 1998). The use of fresh excreta as fertilizer is often combined with the practice to always cook the food and avoid eating raw vegetables, thus reducing potential disease transmission.

In Islamic societies, direct contact with excreta is abhorred; according to Koranic edict, excreta are regarded as containing impurities (*najassa*). Excreta use is permitted only when the *najassa* have been removed (Faruqui, Biswas & Bino, 2001). Thus, the agricultural use of untreated excreta would not be tolerated, and any attempt to modify this view would be futile. On the other hand, excreta use after treatment would be acceptable if the treatment is such that the *najassa* are removed — for example, after thermophilic composting, which produces a humus-like substance that has no visual or odorous connection with the original material. Wastewater may be used for irrigation provided that the impurities (*najassa*) present in the raw wastewater are removed. Untreated wastewater is in fact used in some Islamic countries, principally in areas where there is an extreme water shortage, and then generally from a local wadi (ephemeral desert stream), but this is clearly a result of economic need and not of cultural preference.

In many countries, sanitation facilities that produce fresh excreta, such as bucket latrines, are being replaced by those that do not, such as pour flush toilets. This trend is actively promoted by many governments putting into place pour flush toilets, VIP toilets and urine-diverting toilets. The rationale is not only improved health, but also "society's demand for doing away with the demeaning practice of human beings carrying nightsoil loads" (Venugopalan, 1984). From the viewpoint of excreta-related disease control, this should be welcomed, as the risks to health are substantially reduced. Perceptions about urine are rarely documented, but most people entertain a fairly relaxed attitude towards it. Urine has traditionally been used to smear wounds or as an insecticide to kill banana weevils in East Africa. In contrast to raw faeces, dried and composted faecal material has a distinctly different appearance, similar to ordinary soil, and is more acceptable. It is odourless and has a soil-brown colour that reminds people of soil conditioner. Cultural avoidance of handling well processed composted faecal material is little reported.

Use practices and perceptions of greywater have been little studied. Generally, the view of greywater disposal is relaxed, and little thought is devoted to its management. The interpretation is that the user has been in touch with it in the shower, sink or wash basin before it is discharged, and therefore it might be dirty but not harmful. Greywater contains only minor amounts of faecal excreta, unless diapers have been washed or anal cleansing is practised; it therefore differs from ordinary wastewater and is not regulated by religious edicts.

A common practice in areas with flush toilets where recurring interruptions in water supplies are frequent is the collection by residents of greywater from washing machines and showers to use it for flushing the toilet. In water-scarce areas, residents sometimes unplug greywater taps and use this for watering the garden in periods of restrictions. In parts of India, villagers may bring along the day's greywater to the person who has milk cows as partial payment for the milk (H.C. Sharatchandra, personal communication).

Treated excreta and greywater are much less objectionable in appearance than untreated and from a socioaesthetic viewpoint are more suitable for agricultural use. Therefore, farmers, residents and utilities may take measures to treat or manage urine, faeces and greywater, or a mix of these.

Technical design may minimize contact with and smell or visible aspects of excreta and greywater. Design and technical development of on-site sanitation arrangements can make them odourless, unrecognizable and socioculturally acceptable. Greywater may be discharged in the yard in a mulch bed or subsoil irrigation pipe. Urine may be stored in a tank that is connected to a hose pipe for watering the garden. Faecal matter and toilet paper may be composted.

Generally, farmers seem to have a positive view of the fertilizing value of urine and faecal material, and they may select to use it on crops that are not sensitive to market reactions.

The management structure may have built-in incentives for residents and/or caretakers to fulfil supervision and operational maintenance. There is a need to strike a balance between concealing the system and giving incentives for proper use and sustainability. Use of excreta and greywater can be made safe and acceptable through a combination of technical and management arrangements. The purpose is to have a system that is simple to run well and, ideally, difficult to mismanage. It should be easy to follow the right procedure and difficult to perform the wrong one.

7.2 Food-related determinants

Perceptions of food are related to beliefs, culture, taboos and traditions and are increasingly influenced by mass communication. Food habits are formed under particular social and economic conditions. When adapted to other settings, they may be unsuitable or even harmful to health. For example, rural or indigenous peoples moving to urban areas or migrant workers, tourists or refugees living in foreign communities often maintain their food habits, although the conditions for food production, preparation or processing may be inappropriate or inadequate (WHO, 1995).

The sensory properties of a food item, the anticipated consequences of ingestion and knowledge of the nature or its origin all interact to influence food choice, but the hedonistic response — like or dislike — is the major determinant (WHO, 1995).

7.3 Behavioural change and cultural factors

The rapid growth and increased sophistication of consumer goods from detergents to pharmaceuticals make it increasingly difficult for people to know what they discharge after use. End-of-pipe treatment is not always capable of reducing pollution to acceptable levels and is often expensive. The European Commission is developing a procedure aimed at making manufacturers prove that their products are not harmful to humans or the environment (EU Reach Programme, 2005). This is different from the current administrative system, where the burden of proof of the opposite lies with authorities. To simplify treatment and improve the quality of the resources recovered, separate collection and treatment of different liquid and solid waste streams are commonly practised. In the case of sanitation systems, it generally requires a change in behaviour among the users. Where these changes have occurred, it has been a result of the users' immediate needs and expectations. Attempts to minimize health risks by altering the established excreta use practices are likely to meet with social acceptance and success if the changes are minor and socially unimportant. Any attempts to alter a social preference are likely to fail.

Ingrained routine behaviour may be difficult to change. For instance, it may be hard to abandon the habit of disposing the wastewater of diaper laundry on the lawn if there is no feasible instant alternative for the person doing the washing. However, as is often the case, a simple technical improvement such as letting the water run into a mulch bed can help to solve the potential contamination problem.

Studies of alternative sanitation in housing areas show that residents may be willing to take on new responsibilities for environmental reasons. Among users, criteria such as privacy, convenience, cost and ease of construction or maintenance are, however, often considered more important in system selection than the protection of human health or the environment (Guzha & Musara, 2004; Holden, Terreblanche & Muller, 2004). The absence of flies and odour in correctly maintained urine diversion toilets and their permanent structures, allowing them to be built directly onto a house, have proven to be important factors in their widespread use in areas of South Africa, where they are seen as a modern sanitation alternative (Drangert, 2004a).

Behavioural change regarding toilet use has occurred rapidly when local conditions have created an imperative for the recovery and use of excreta and/or greywater (Wirbelauer, Breslin & Guzha, 2003), such as a need for improved sanitation or for the products, such as fertilizer, soil conditioner or biogas. Physical conditions, such as high water table, regular flooding as well as rocky areas with high cost for digging trenches in the area, may prevent conventional sanitation solutions; instead, dry urine-diverting toilets may represent an affordable alternative to improve sanitation. For coastal estuaries as well as waterlogged areas occupied by the urban poor, technically sound and socially acceptable solutions may be found. In dry areas with poor soils, use of greywater and treated excreta may become a driving force for improved sanitation, since application will make urban agriculture possible, as has been demonstrated in West Africa.

Improved public health should always be combined with promoting better domestic and personal hygiene through education and behavioural change. In excreta use systems, the people most at risk are those who apply the excreta to the fields, their families, produce handlers, consumers of produce and people with access to the areas where excreta are used (Kochar, 1979). There is a whole range of behaviours that can be targeted to better protect public health.

Improving sanitation facilities and convincing people to use them properly are the first step. It is also important to demonstrate the public health benefits of adequately treating or storing excreta before its use as fertilizer. Information for residents and farmers has a better chance to be effective if it provides "facts" about what will happen if advice is followed and if they receive feedback on routine changes. The information provider should make sure that the focus is on effective measures to achieve the stated purpose and to do this "right thing" in the right way (efficiency).

Educational efforts can be directed at school children — for example, informing them about helminth infections, their life cycles and preventive measures against transmission. Encouraging workers to use protective gear (e.g. rubber boots and gloves) while harvesting or handling crops/products will reduce exposure to infectious agents, and improving hygienic practices (handwashing!) during produce handling, transport and produce preparation for consumption is very important. Communities should educate people about the risks associated with contact with untreated excreta. Direct work with farmers to restrict the types of produce grown in excreta-fertilized fields is advocated.

In many cases, it will be possible to tie efforts to achieve hygienic behavioural changes through education to ongoing agricultural extension and health outreach activities (Blumenthal et al., 2000). However, health interventions should focus on a few key specific behaviours to be successful and may work better if social and cultural reasons for changing hygienic practices are emphasized rather than motivation building on health benefits (Curtis & Kanki, 1998; Blumenthal et al., 2000). The acceptance of a change in sanitary practices is facilitated when users have been given the opportunity to examine and identify their own problems and are offered a wider choice of sanitation systems. "Seeing is believing" has also proved important in overcoming reservations concerning the use of certain systems, particularly when people have had the opportunity to visit them in the homes of neighbours or peers. The equipment and treatment used, the necessary maintenance and the recycled resources available and their form have to be both economically affordable and socially and culturally acceptable. This can best be achieved with the active participation of all relevant stakeholders in planning processes, as is conceived by the PHAST method (see section 11.2.1; WHO, UNDP & WSP, 1997; WHO, 2004a).

The willingness of communities and individuals to collect, treat and use greywater and excreta varies enormously from one country to another, and also within societies. Where poor farming households lack access to fertilizers, the use of excreta in agriculture is often well known and acceptable, but when civil servants working in cities are presented with the concept, these may have difficulty accepting it, often supported by their argument that the people who are expected to apply it would not accept it.

7.4 Convenience factors and dignity issues

Convenient use and operation have proven to be of crucial importance for users of sanitation facilities, including the level of comfort, privacy and security. The cost to construct and maintain installations is another important consideration. Many users who have changed to urine-diverting systems from pit or VIP latrines appreciate the level of comfort that, by their perception, is comparable with that of water toilets. When permanently installed in the house, they are more convenient for use day and night and provide security for women and girls who would otherwise be exposed to the risk of sexual harassment when visiting external toilet facilities. Permanent in-house structures receive a great deal of attention and have therefore become status symbols in some areas. They can also be adapted to accommodate different anal cleansing practices (Drangert, 2004a).

One of the greatest perceived inconveniences of these systems is the need for handling of faeces. During this activity, the exposure should be minimized. It has implications for the esteem that the community at large attributes to those engaged in it. In some parts of southern Africa, the practice of collecting and using someone else's excreta is looked upon unfavourably. However, an example from South Africa shows that with the right economic incentives, it may be acceptable (Drangert, 2006). In this case, a contractor collects the dry faeces and is paid by the residents for this service. The residents view him as a service provider. He, in turn, runs a successful company, recovering the nutrients and selling the treated product back to the residents.

The handling of excreta is closely linked to issues of human dignity. In some societies, those working with excreta or wastewater may be perceived as "unclean," and the work is often a task reserved for those living on the margins of society in the weakest of social positions. One example of this can be seen among the Dhalits in India, although most states have outlawed the concept since the 1980s. One of the jobs assigned to them is the manual disposal of human excreta. For conventional sanitation systems, a similar handling of fresh, untreated faeces or wastewater may pose a risk to the health of workers in this area. This may involve emptying buckets or pits or unblocking sewage networks, frequently without appropriate protective clothing. Systems aimed at using on-site treatment approaches for excreta may reduce exposures to untreated faeces and create better conditions for those working in sanitation.

The privacy and convenience of the urine-diverting sanitation installations are often seen as protecting and promoting human dignity, by providing safe, private toilet facilities. Care should be taken in the design to ensure not only that they meet the needs of the majority of the adult population but also that sanitation facilities are accessible and usable for small children, the elderly and the disabled, and that their dignity is protected. In-house facilities can help to ensure that these goals are achieved.

7.5 Gender aspects on use of excreta and greywater

While men in most areas construct latrines, women are usually responsible for keeping them clean and usable. Women assist children, the aged and the sick with their hygiene and sanitation needs. Women also take responsibility for teaching children about the use of latrines and providing them with health/hygiene education. Women's perceptions, needs and priorities in relation to sanitation are therefore quite different from men's. Safety (particularly for children) and privacy appear to be the main concerns of women. What men want in relation to sanitation has never been specifically assessed. Men's interests, needs and priorities in relation to sanitation may well be as neglected as women's.

In parts of India, open defecation forces women and girls to enter the demarcated area for defecation outside the village. They are vulnerable to abuse or rape, particularly in the evening. Their choice is often to either use a "pottie" in the house or refrain until morning. Fathers are protective of the girls and prevent pre-marriage affairs, but this does not appear to be a compelling factor for installing a toilet in the house. There is no outspoken societal norm requesting men to do so, despite the fact that their daughter may be hurt. This highlights the need to translate the male task of constructing toilets into a non-negotiable social norm.

Another indication of deviation from male responsibility in East Africa (Drangert, 2004b) relates to the choice of locating the urine-diverting toilet inside the house or in the backyard. Male heads of households often opt to have the toilet in the yard, while female heads prefer that the toilet be indoors. This reflects the perceived benefits of the indoor toilet for women's household chores, while men tend to undervalue female benefits and talk instead about the risk of a bad odour. Also, men generally have more options for excreting; they work outside the home more often and can use the facilities at the workplace or elsewhere. The gender perspectives on sanitation systems that intentionally recover and use excreta and greywater have not yet been specifically explored. Women are actively involved in food crop production and concerned about food security. They would be directly affected by increased access to soil nutrients provided by such systems. Access to a ready supply of fertilizer will help to increase food production and facilitate the development of small vegetable gardens and fruit trees close to homes.

Given women's overall prime responsibility for the health and well-being of families in many areas, it may also be assumed that they would support such systems on the basis of health gains. Women's support would also be critical for the success of different methods to treat faeces and ensure a sufficient reduction in pathogens. Since women have the responsibility for tending the cooking fires, their involvement could be used to ensure a supply of ashes to be used in the latrines. Men construct the latrine, and it may be assumed that they would appreciate not having to construct a new latrine and pit each time the old pit is filled. The possibility of simply emptying the toilet chamber and continuing to use it must be positive from a labour expenditure point of view. However, this task has to be done on a regular basis, which makes it different from typically male household tasks. Both women and men need access to cash incomes and would be assumed to welcome the potential economic benefits of excreta and greywater use, if the opportunities for small-scale entrepreneurship in construction of sanitation facilities and starting small market gardens are made available to both women and men. In India, the fertilizer value of a family's excreta can pay for the investment in a urine diversion toilet within four years (Jönsson et al., 2005).

It has long been established that lack of access to adequate sanitation facilities, in particular from a privacy perspective, has implications for the education of girls. Parents are reluctant to send their girls to school in some parts of the world where school sanitation is inadequate. Experience from Tanzania in the 1980s revealed that parents sometimes took their girls out of primary school altogether because of poor sanitation facilities. In other cases, girls' schooling was irregular because inadequate facilities did not permit them to go to school during menstruation. Such systems can therefore contribute to the schooling of girls by providing access to appropriate and adequate sanitation.

Women retain most of the sanitary tasks for cleaning the latrine or toilet in the home. They are often involved in gardening and responsible for feeding the family. Therefore, the potential use of urine and greywater in fertilizing and watering the garden — be it a lawn, trees or vegetables — does not require a change of responsibilities between men and women in the household. By contributing to urban agriculture, treated excreta and greywater could help families save money by growing their own fruit and vegetables and/or selling some of the produce. Women often have a great need for increased sources of income but are often confined to the informal sector. Urban agriculture, as a means of ensuring greater food security and potential supplementary income, is particularly attractive to women, as it allows them to work close to their homes and facilitates the carrying out of other important roles, such as care of children, elderly and the sick. The importance of ensuring that women, as well as men, are involved in planning and decision-making on urban agriculture initiatives and have equitable access to training and extension services deserves special attention.

In areas with high water tables in South India, where other forms of sanitation are not feasible, sanitation systems that facilitate excreta and greywater use provide advantage for to women and girls. Without access to sanitation, the alternative for poor households is that all members of the households have to walk to open defecation sites (separate sites for women and men), sometimes at a distance of up to 0.5 km from the household. The health risks at the defecation sites are considerable. There are additional problems for women and girls, as they are able to use these sites to urinate and defecate only at dawn and dusk. The toilet in use in South India requires much less water than the more expensive alternative, the water flush toilets, which reduces the work burden for women in drawing and carrying water for the toilets.

Experience from Zimbabwe (Morgan, 2005) indicates that women in rural areas prefer the sanitation alternative offered by the arbour loos (an "arbour loo" is a simple form of latrine with a shallow pit, with a light, moveable slab. When the pit is three quarters full, a new pit is dug, and the slab and superstructure are moved to the new site. The old one is covered with topsoil, in which a fruit tree is planted) to the conventional pit latrines, as they can be built closer to the house. Women expressed appreciation of the gains in terms of privacy and safety, particularly for children, in night use. Women also consider the use of the filled pits for planting fruit trees beneficial. Having the fruit trees close to the house enhances the potential for tending them properly, particularly in terms of being able to use the greywater from bathing and dish washing for watering. Men expressed appreciation of the arbour loos because the pits are smaller than conventional pit latrines and building them requires less labour. These findings are, however, based not on well documented empirical data but on the observation of practitioners working in the communities.

When sanitation alternatives are being considered, it should be ensured that women are involved in all decision-making processes, even if traditionally they are excluded from decisions seen as being outside of the family, connected with the allocation of finances or concerned with "technical measures." It should be remembered that if these systems fail, women would usually be the group most severely affected.

Addressing gender issues implies taking a closer look at social structure and relationships between women and men and between girls and boys and examining the different roles of community members. Considering gender is therefore not just a matter of involving women in a sanitation project; the first goal is to make gender roles and interdependencies visible and to include this in the implementation process. The roles of men and women with regard to decision-making, choice of technology, hygiene, food security, financial security, crop production and health issues should be determined in order to involve the correct groups in an appropriate, participatory manner (Werner et al., 2003).

8
ENVIRONMENTAL ASPECTS

The use of excreta and greywater in agriculture has the potential for both positive and negative environmental impacts. The resource value of excreta and greywater has been largely described in chapter 1. The present chapter reviews the potential environmental impacts associated with the use of urine, faeces and greywater, which will differ depending on local conditions.

It is important to minimize the environmental impact associated with the direct use of excreta and greywater in agriculture in both the local and global context. For large-scale implementation, environmental impact assessment is a useful tool for the analysis. A procedure for measuring the environmental impacts of different sanitation approaches involves the analysis of material flows (see case study in Box 8.1) or a life cycle analysis for the production of different crops, which may also lead to a better understanding of the environmental impacts of different agricultural practices (see case study in Box 8.2).

Box 8.1 Example of environmental assessment through material flow analysis

A case study conducted in Viet Tri, Viet Nam, allowed an estimation of nitrogen flows related to excreta and organic solid waste management in Viet Tri by applying the method of material flow analysis (Montangero, Nguyen & Belevi, 2004). The results indicate that 60% of the nitrogen delivered to the households in the form of food is finally discharged with the excreta in surface water, in fish ponds or on the soil, resulting in water pollution. The impact of potential control measures — including increasing the proportion of households using urine diversion latrines from 5% to 25%, treating 25% of the effluent from on-site sanitation systems in duckweed ponds and treating 25% of the sludge from on-site systems in constructed wetlands — was quantified. The proposed measures led to a 30% reduction of the nitrogen load into soil and surface water.

Box 8.2 Life cycle analysis of wheat production using human urine as fertilizer

Life cycle analysis is another tool for monitoring environmental sustainability. The environmental consequences of introducing urine as a fertilizer for cereals were studied by Tidåker (2003). Conventional production of spring barley with a chemical fertilizer was compared with the same production using urine as fertilizer. If the collection system and handling were optimized and well functioning, the energy use decreased by 27% when urine was used as fertilizer. Eutrophication of surface waters was substantially lowered due to lower discharge of nitrogen and phosphorus, but a higher release of ammonia to the atmosphere occurred. The environmental impact depended on decisions made at the farm level, highlighting the need for monitoring the reuse system from the toilet all the way to the field.

The environmental impact of different sanitation systems can be measured in terms of the use of natural resources, discharges to water bodies, air emissions and impacts on soils. Table 8.1 summarizes the types of impacts that may be considered in an environmental impact assessment (Kvarnström et al., 2004). Most relevant in relation to the use of excreta and greywater are the potential environmental impacts on soil and water bodies.

8.1 Impacts on soil

Relevant substances to consider in terms of environmental impacts on soil are salts, heavy metals, persistent organic compounds, hormones and nutrients.

8.1.1 Metals

The content of heavy metals in excreta is generally low or very low, compared with other sources with potential impacts on soil, and depends on the amounts present in consumed food products. The contents of urine reflect metabolism, and the levels of heavy metals in urine are very low (Jönsson et al., 1999; Vinnerås, 2002; Palmquist, 2004). Concentrations of heavy metals are relatively higher in faeces than in urine, but the concentrations are lower than in chemical fertilizers (e.g. cadmium) and farmyard manure (e.g. chromium and lead). The main proportion of the micronutrients and other heavy metals passes through the intestine unaffected (Fraústo da Silva & Williams, 1997). Of all the liquid household effluents, greywater may have the highest heavy metal content.

Table 8.1 Criteria for measuring environmental impacts of sanitation systems

Criteria	Unit
Use of natural resources, construction, operation and maintenance	
Land	m^2/person
Energy	MJ/person
Construction materials	Type and volume
Chemicals	Type and volume
Fresh water	m^3/person per year
Discharge to water bodies	
BOD/COD	g/person per year
Impact on eutrophication	g/person per year of nitrogen and phosphorus
Hazardous substances: heavy metals, persistent organic compounds, pharmaceutical residues, hormones, pathogens	mg/person per year; number/unit
Air emissions	
Contribution to global warming	kg of carbon dioxide equivalents
Resources recovered	
Nutrients	% into the system
Energy	% consumption within the system
Organic materials	% into the system
Water	% into the system
Quality of recycled product released to soil	
Hazardous substances: heavy metals, persistent organic compounds, pharmaceutical residues, hormones, pathogens	mg/unit; number/unit

Source: Kvarnström et al. (2004).

Regardless of the metal content of the excreta and greywater, a metal will not impact plant uptake unless it first reaches a threshold concentration in the soil and the metal is in a mobile phase (i.e. dissolved in the soil solution and not adsorbed to soil particles). Metals are bound to soils at a pH above 6.5 and/or with high organic matter content. If the pH is below this value, organic matter is consumed or all feasible soil adsorption sites are saturated, metals become mobile and can be absorbed by crops and contaminate water bodies. The plant roots act as an efficient barrier against uptake of non-essential metals. Therefore, impacts on soils from heavy metals are usually noted on soil microbiology before they are observed in plants or ultimately humans (or animals). Impacts of heavy metals on crops are complex, because there humans (or animals). Impacts of heavy metals on crops are complex, because there may be antagonistic interactions that affect their uptake by plants (Drakatos et al., 2002).

One important heavy metal is cadmium, which is a non-essential element that can pass through the root barrier, due to its resemblance to zinc. Cadmium is toxic to humans and needs to be limited in the inflow to agricultural land. Heavy metal concentrations in excreta and greywater generated at the household or small community level will rarely be high enough, however, to threaten the environment.

Table 8.2 Concentrations of heavy metals in urine, faeces, wastewater and source-diverted kitchen waste, compared with farmyard manure

	Unit	Cu	Zn	Cr	Ni	Pb	Cd
Urine	µg/kg ww	67	30	7	5	1	0
Faeces	µg/kg ww	6 667	65 000	122	450	122	62
Blackwater	µg/kg ww	716	6 420	18	49	13	7
Kitchen waste	µg/kg ww	6 837	8 717	1 706	1 025	3 425	34
Cattle organic farmyard manure	µg/kg ww	5 220	26 640	684	630	184	23
Urine	mg/kg P	101	45	10	7	2	1
Faeces	mg/kg P	2 186	21 312	40	148	40	20
Blackwater	mg/kg P	797	7 146	20	54	15	7
Kitchen waste	mg/kg P	5 279	6 731	1 317	791	2 644	26
Sewage sludge	mg/kg P	13 360	19 793	1 072	617	1 108	46.9
Cattle organic farmyard manure	mg/kg P	3 537	18 049	463	427	124	16

ww: wet weight
Sources: Steineck et al. (1999); Vinnerås (2002).

8.1.2 Persistent organic compounds

Excreta and greywater normally have low contents of persistent organic compounds. However, depending on the household use, greywater may contain as many as 900 different organic compounds; nevertheless, most of these substances will be found at very low concentrations (Eriksson et al., 2002). Collected faecal sludge may also contain a range of different organic chemicals used in the household if they have been dumped in the toilet. Information to system users regarding the importance of correct handling of household chemicals is vital.

If excreta and greywater are treated prior to use in agriculture, the concentration of many of these compounds will be reduced by adsorption, volatilization and biodegradation. Absorption of these substances by plants through their root system is not likely to occur due to their usually large size and high molecular weight, which reduces their mobility in soil and water (Pahren et al., 1979). It is possible that these chemicals can be transferred to the edible surfaces of crops, but concentrations are likely to be low. These substances may be associated with soil that remains on the crops after harvest. Washing produce thoroughly prior to consumption will remove a large percentage of this contamination.

Synthetic organic compounds are adsorbed and biodegraded with time in soil. Cordy et al. (2003) studied the removal of 34 organic compounds that can be found in excreta and greywater and did not detect any of them after 3 m of infiltration through desert soils with a retention time of 21 days. Removal of endocrine disruptors such as steroidal hormones detected in treated and non-treated wastewater through infiltration in soils has been demonstrated (Mansell, Drewes & Rauch, 2004).

A variety of pharmaceutical residues or their metabolic by-products can be detected in excreta and sometimes greywater. Most of these substances are at the highest concentrations in urine. A number of biologically active pharmaceuticals and their metabolites have been identified in groundwater and drinking-water samples (Heberer, Schmidt-Bäumler & Stan, 1998; Heberer, 2002). The effects of these substances on the ecosystem and animals are not known, but negative effects on the quantity or quality of crops are assumed to be negligible. Furthermore, the amount of hormones in manure from domestic animals is far greater than the amount found in human urine or faeces. Thus, even though theoretical estimates based on effects on fish have indicated an ecotoxicological effect from estradiol, comparative assessments with manure strongly indicate that the risk is very limited (Hanselman, Graetz & Wilkie, 2003).

Urine and faecal fertilizers are mixed into the topsoil, where there is a high level of biological activity. Usually the substances are retained there for months. The dominant removal mechanism for these substances is adsorption. Removal efficiencies are greater in soils containing higher contents of silt, clay and organic matter. Some may be transported through the soil matrix to groundwater, and two drugs (carbamazepine and primidone) did not show significant reductions even after six years of passage through the soil aquifer treatment system (Drewes, Heberer & Reddersen, 2002). Additional attenuation, to below the detection limit, occurs by biodegradation, regardless of aerobic or anoxic conditions or the type of organic carbon matrix present (hydrophobic acids, hydrophilic carbon vs colloidal carbon). A variety of pharmaceutical residues or their metabolic by-products in low concentrations can be detected in wastewater, which may reflect either that they are excreted in urine and faeces or that they are flushed away in the toilet.

Endocrine disruptors (which interfere with hormone functions) have also been found in greywater and may not degrade quickly in the environment. Mansell, Drewes & Rauch (2004) found that 17-α-estradiol, estriol and testosterone are not sensitive to photodegradation (i.e. less than 10% destruction after 24-h exposure to ultraviolet light). Thus, these compounds could remain on the surface of crops irrigated with greywater that contains them. The concentrations of these compounds are usually extremely low, and to date only effects on animals in direct contact with polluted water have been demonstrated. Effects on humans have not been shown.

Regarding excreta, some substances with endocrine disrupting properties, such as hormones (from humans, e.g. 7-ethinylestradiol, or from plants, e.g. 17-α-estradiol estriol) and pharmaceuticals, may be present in low concentrations, especially in diverted urine. It should be noted that animal manure also contains residues of pharmaceuticals used, in many cases preventive medication, resulting in high amounts of, especially, antibiotics. The soil system is generally better equipped than watercourses for degradation of the pharmaceutical residues present in the fertilizers.

8.1.3 Salinization

Salinity effects are, in general, of concern only in arid and semi-arid regions, where accumulated salts are not flushed regularly from the soil profile by rainfall. The use of urine and greywater can accelerate the process of soil salinization due to its higher salt content. However, fertilizers containing organic materials will help to buffer the negative effects of the salts in the soil profile.

There are four ways in which salinity affects soil productivity:

1) It changes the osmotic pressure at the root zone.
2) It provokes specific ion (sodium, boron or chloride) toxicity.
3) It may interfere with plant uptake of essential nutrients (e.g. potassium and nitrate) due to antagonism with sodium, chloride and sulfates.
4) It may destroy the soil structure by causing soil dispersion and clogging of pore spaces. This results in an increased lateral drainage, but may also affect the oxygenation. Both low-salinity waters and high sodium concentrations in the water in relation to calcium and magnesium concentrations in the soil exacerbate the effects.

Salinization is measured through a combination of parameters. Depending on the type of soils and the washing and drainage conditions, salinity problems can occur with conductivities of >3 mS/m, dissolved solids concentrations of >500 mg/l (being severe if >2000 mg/l) and sodium adsorption ratios of >3–9 (Ayers & Westcott, 1985). Soil salinization is also affected by inefficient drainage, climate and type of soil. Practices to limit salinization include soil washing and appropriate soil drainage.

8.2 Impacts on water bodies

Application of excreta and greywater to agricultural land will reduce the direct impacts on water bodies. However, as for any type of fertilizer, the nutrients may percolate to groundwater if applied in excess or be flushed into surface water after excessive rainfall. This impact will always be less compared with that of the direct use of water bodies as the primary recipient.

The impact of reuse of human excreta and greywater in agriculture on groundwater quality depends on factors such as agricultural application rate, the type of irrigation water, the soil type, aquifer vulnerability, the agricultural practices and the type of crops, as well as the recharge and groundwater use (Foster et al., 2004).

In order to avoid negative effects of using excreta and greywater as agricultural fertilizers, the following should be considered (Foster et al., 2004):

- improve agricultural practices;
- establish criteria to operate wells used to supply water for human consumption in the surroundings (establish safe distances to the agricultural site, depth of extraction and appropriate construction);
- routinely monitor groundwater.

Surface water bodies are affected by agricultural drainage and runoff. Impacts depend on the type of water body (rivers, agricultural channels, lakes or dams) and their use, as well as the hydraulic retention time and their function within the ecosystem.

A high organic load will, independently of the source, affect the dissolved oxygen levels, thus impacting aquatic organisms. Additionally, the nitrogen or phosphorus washed into water bodies will lead to eutrophication and subsequent oxygen depletion and will facilitate the growth of toxin-producing algae (Chorus & Bartram, 1999).

Organic chemicals originating from excreta and greywater will only minimally impact surface water bodies due to their adsorption to soil particles after application. The soil will act as a filter before the respective pollutants reach groundwater and surface waters.

Nitrogen can contaminate groundwater and surface water bodies by infiltration and agricultural runoff. The amount of nitrogen leached depends on crop demand, hydraulic load due to rain and agricultural water, soil permeability and nitrogen content in soils. Agricultural runoff containing phosphorus can cause eutrophication in surface water bodies (reservoirs and lakes). High concentrations of biodegradable organic matter in agricultural runoff water can lead to the consumption of dissolved oxygen in lakes and rivers.

Phosphorus is an essential element for plant growth, and mined phosphates are a common input into agricultural production in order to increase crop productivity. Soil phosphorus content varies with parent material, texture and management factors, such as rate of application, type of phosphorus applied and soil cultivation (Sharpley, 1995). It is usually present in soils in relatively important quantities. World supplies of accessible mined phosphate are diminishing. It is predicted that phosphate-carrying rocks/mineral reserves will run out in 60–130 years. The mining of phosphate causes environmental damage because it is often removed close to the surface in large open mines, leaving behind scarred land. Moreover, phosphate-carrying rocks/minerals also contain varying amounts of non-desired elements, such as cadmium. Approximately 25% of the mined phosphorus ends up in aquatic environments or buried in landfills or other sinks (Tiessen, 1995). The discharge into aquatic environments causes eutrophication of water bodies, leading to more environmental damage. To reduce the phenomenon of eutrophication, wastewater treatment plants require additional phosphorus removal treatment capacity, which adds to the costs and complexity of the treatment process.

Urine alone contains more than 50% of the phosphorus excreted by humans. Thus, the diversion of urine and its use in agriculture can aid crop production and reduce the need for costly, advanced wastewater treatment processes to remove phosphorus from the effluents (EcoSanRes, 2005).

9
ECONOMIC AND FINANCIAL CONSIDERATIONS

Economic factors are especially important when the viability of a new scheme for the use of excreta and greywater in agriculture is assessed, but even an economically worthwhile project can fail without careful financial planning.

Economic analysis and financial considerations are critical underpinnings for the promotion of the safe use of excreta and greywater. Economic analysis seeks to establish the economic feasibility of a proposed project in a broad macroeconomic context and allows economic comparisons between different options to implement the project. The costs transferred to other sectors — for example, as a result of health and environmental impacts on downstream communities — also should be included as distinct components in a cost analysis. This can be achieved through multiple-objective decision-making processes.

Financial planning looks at how the project is to be paid for. In establishing the financial feasibility of a project, it is important to determine the sources and flows of revenue and to clarify who will pay for what. The ability to profitably market the treated greywater and excreta or the products grown with them also needs analysis. Market feasibility assessment is discussed in section 9.3.

9.1 Economic feasibility

Economics looks at the optimal use of limited resources and at opportunities foregone by their use. In the context of excreta and greywater use for agriculture, economic analyses seek to establish whether resources invested in such projects have optimal returns, bearing in mind the resource value of excreta and greywater themselves. There are a number of methods that can be used to economically analyse projects, with cost-effectiveness analysis and cost–benefit analysis being the most important. The availability of reliable data sets and the setting of realistic and meaningful boundaries critically determine the quality of economic evaluations.

9.1.1 Cost–benefit analysis

Cost-effectiveness analysis has been frequently used for the economic evaluation of different health intervention options, offsetting costs against agreed, meaningful health indicators. Outside the health sector, planners are accustomed to cost–benefit analysis. Within the framework of a cost–benefit analysis, monetary values are assigned to all expected costs and benefits of a project. This allows decisions on whether and how to do projects, based on the internal rate of return. The introduction of the DALY as a composite measure of community health has made it possible to apply cost–benefit analyses to health interventions in an intersectoral context, such as is the case for the safe use of excreta and greywater in agriculture. The economic appraisal of an excreta and greywater use project is undertaken to determine the efficiency of the project, as a basis to decide whether it is worthwhile to proceed with it (Squire & van der Tak, 1975; Gittinger, 1982). This requires a calculation of the marginal costs and benefits of the project — that is, the differences between the costs and benefits of the project and the costs and benefits of the alternative. For any scheme to be economically viable, its marginal benefits should exceed its marginal costs.

The strength of cost–benefit analyses of sanitation schemes lies in the production of comparable data for a range of different sanitation options as a basis for decision-making. The comprehensiveness of the cost analysis component is critical, and it should therefore explicitly include direct costs related to the system hardware and software components, but also indirect costs incurred by other components, such as planning, administration, hygiene promotion campaigns and the health and environmental impacts on downstream communities.

9.1.2 Costs and benefits

Traditional economic evaluations of sanitation systems tend to face an important hurdle: the definition of the system boundaries often leads to substantial costs and/or benefits being completely overlooked. How substantial these costs can actually be becomes apparent from the example of a centralized wastewater treatment plant that discharges treated effluent to a surface water body. In addition to the investment, reinvestment and operation and maintenance costs of the sewer network and treatment plant, costs incurred by the environmental problems arising in the receiving water should be considered, as should those of the social loss of a recreational area, of the possible effect on subsequent drinking-water treatment, of the loss of natural habitats, of effects on coastal areas and of using drinking-water to flush the system. Each one of these indirect costs may in turn incur further costs.

For systems using excreta and greywater, the indirect costs may include those of the necessary transformation to adapt the existing sanitary infrastructure, additional awareness-raising activities to ensure its proper use and the need for continued research and development of the system.

For a centralized wastewater treatment facility, the expected health benefits for those connected to the system are obvious. The safe use of excreta and greywater has a number of indirect benefits to be considered, including:

- preserving high-quality water sources for priority uses, such as drinking-water supply (through the possible use of treated greywater for irrigation water and by not discharging effluents to water sources);
- an improvement of soil structure and fertility;
- increased access to fertilizer, particularly for poor subsistence farmers (thus increasing harvests and food security);
- reduced energy consumption (both in the treatment works and for fertilizer production);
- possible energy production and resource conservation;
- creation of small- and medium-sized businesses, selling technologies or services associated with the collection, treatment and/or marketing of the products.

It is therefore essential that economic evaluations comparing these two options be of a sufficiently strategic nature and that they take into account economies of scale in decentralized systems.

Further economic and financial considerations guiding the choice of sanitation systems for the safe use of excreta and greywater include the following:

- Sewerage systems are expensive to build, operate and maintain — systems that can reduce the infrastructure needs (e.g. on-site dry sanitation, with or without urine diversion) may be much less expensive.
- The cost of pumping greywater or transporting excreta can be substantial — greywater and excreta treatment facilities should be planned where the greywater and excreta can be efficiently used with minimal transport (e.g. neighbourhood biogas digestors could be used to treat excreta from on-site systems in urban areas).
- Effective low-cost greywater and excreta treatment technologies are available.
- Combinations of different treatment technologies (e.g. composting toilets plus post-composting with organic material) may increase pathogen removal

efficiencies at low cost and provide flexibility for upgrading treatment facilities.
- Users of greywater and excreta may be willing to pay for the greywater and excreta.
- Greywater and excreta tariffs may help to foster cost recovery, and the sale of crops at a central facility may also raise revenues.
- Differential prices for treated greywater and excreta and freshwater or agricultural inputs may entice farmers to use greywater and excreta instead of high-quality freshwater sources or expensive imported fertilizers.

Excreta and greywater use systems can influence the economic status at the household level and at the national level. If excreta and greywater are treated and managed properly, health risks are significantly reduced. At the household level, the resources spent on caring for or curing a sick person may be allocated to other tasks, and time gained through reduced illness can be used for education or income-generating activities. At the national level, the burden on scarce financial and human resources in the health sector may be reduced and can be realloted to other areas.

9.1.3 Multiple-objective decision-making processes

The information produced by economic evaluations helps support decision-making processes, but it should be combined with information that allows other factors and externalities to be taken into account. To be able to objectively compare different sanitation systems, there is a need for fully integrated cost–benefit or multiple-criteria analyses of all types of sanitation systems, performed over system life cycles or planning periods. This can be achieved using multiple-objective decision-making approaches. These involve establishing criteria that consider all key aspects of the system (e.g. health, environmental, sociocultural, economic and technical aspects) and using these to form a basis for decision-making.

A range of different quantification methods can be used in multiple-criteria approaches outside of estimated monetary values, with DALYs as a measure of health effects and various measurable indicators (e.g. the use of natural resources, discharge to water bodies, etc.) for the environment. Sociocultural aspects, such as the appropriateness of the system or its legal acceptability, can be qualitatively assessed, as can technical issues, such as system robustness or its compatibility with existing systems. The analysis of a specific proposed project should involve not only a comparison of one system with another, but also a comparison of the options to implement one particular scheme — for instance, the use of greywater for different purposes (irrigation, industrial, non-potable uses).

9.1.4 Empirical examples of cost analyses for reuse systems

One of the difficulties in the economic evaluation of sanitation systems that promote the use of excreta and greywater is that very few studies have so far been carried out and that when information is available, it is mainly from pilot or demonstration projects, which have additional expenses (e.g. for technology introduction costs, limited, small-scale fabrication of system elements, awareness-raising activities, etc.). Such studies have also tended to consider only a particular aspect of the system rather than adopt a holistic view. Studies that have considered only investment, reinvestment and operation and maintenance costs have shown, however, that systems designed to use excreta and greywater have a financial advantage over more conventional systems (see Box 9.1).

Box 9.1 Examples of investment and operation and maintenance cost comparisons

Germany

In Brandenburg, near Berlin, Germany, cost comparisons have been made for three different sanitation concepts for a planned new housing estate, where the population is expected to increase from 672 to 5000 inhabitants within 10 years. The three systems analysed were:

1) *Conventional*: Gravity sewer system, consisting of flush toilets, conventional gravity sewer system, pumping station with transport sewer to the existing sewer network, system operated by the public supplier.
2) *Gravity*: Source separation concept I (gravity, composting of faeces), consisting of gravity separation toilets, collection and storage of urine, transport and agricultural use on a nearby farm, faeces transported in gravity sewer with aerobic treatment in a compost separator, utilization of compost in horticulture, transport of greywater in gravity sewer system, treatment in a constructed wetland, transport to the receiving water body.
3) *Vacuum*: Source separation concept II (vacuum, digestion of faeces), consisting of vacuum separation toilets, gravity urine transport, storage of the urine and agricultural use on a nearby farm, faeces transported by vacuum sewerage, common treatment with organic waste in a biogas plant, biogas used to produce energy, transport of the digested sludge to nearby farms and utilization in agriculture, transport of greywater in gravity sewer system, treatment in a constructed wetland, transport to the receiving water.

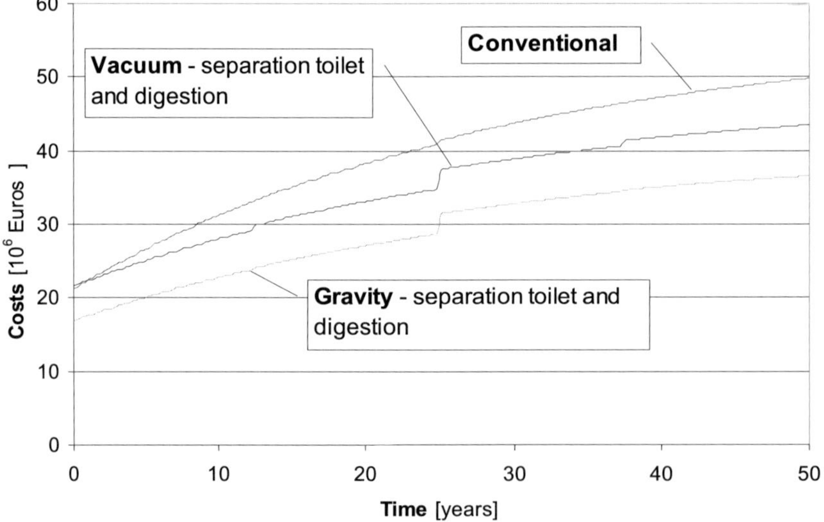

Figure 9.1

Cost comparison for the installation, operation and maintenance of the three systems for a population of 5000 in Brandenburg, Germany

The costs associated with the three systems were calculated over a lifetime of 50 years, with an annual interest rate of 3.5% per annum. The results of this cost comparison can be clearly seen in Figure 9.1, for the situation where 5000 inhabitants are served and the local Berlin water company is responsible for the operation of the system. Other service scenarios have been calculated with different population numbers and operational models, which also revealed a significant price advantage for the use-oriented systems over the system's lifetime.

Box 9.1 (continued)

Uganda

In Kalungu Girls Secondary School in Uganda, existing sanitation facilities were posing a risk to groundwater quality, the main source of potable water. In 2003, a project was implemented to renew and improve both water supply and sanitation facilities at the school. Additionally, a training programme aimed at ensuring an understanding and proper use of the new facilities was implemented.

Prior to deciding on the sanitation scheme, a detailed cost comparison was conducted and served as one instrument in the decision-making progress. Two alternative sanitary solutions were compared:

1) *Option 1: Source separation concept*: Dry urine diversion toilets, sewer line for greywater and a horizontal subsurface flow constructed wetland. The treated products from the toilets are to be used to water gardens within the school grounds.
2) *Option 2: Conventional concept*: Flush toilets for the students, separate sewer system for wastewater, mechanical pretreatment, pumping station and a vertical subsurface flow constructed wetland.

The comparison considered investment and reinvestment and operating costs. The calculation was carried out over a 50-year time frame, with reinvestments depending on individual system parts and an interest rate of 8% per annum.

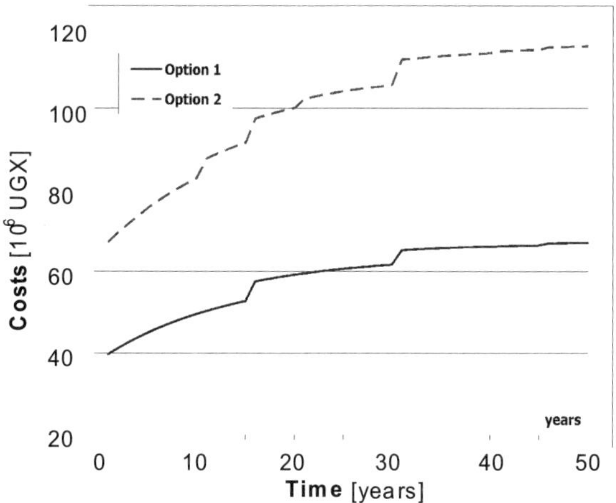

Figure 9.2

Cost comparison for the installation, operation and maintenance of the two systems for the school (exchange rate as of 22 September 2004: 1€ = 2060 UGX).

The cost comparison in Figure 9.2 shows that the safe use option is significantly less expensive. The main difference results from the significantly smaller wastewater treatment system for this option and the pumping station required for the conventional option.

9.2 Financial feasibility

To ensure sustainable services and cost recovery of excreta and greywater use systems, appropriate financing mechanisms are needed. A financial cost analysis should consider not only the investment, reinvestment and operation and maintenance requirements of the system, but also the indirect costs as well as the system's impacts on the environment, individuals and communities (Cardone & Fonseca, 2003).

Funds will be needed to ensure institutional capacity building and skills development, assessment and monitoring, policy formulation and the creation of an enabling environment for sanitation. The latter includes awareness-raising campaigns, hygiene promotion, public consultations and hearings, and informing policy- and decision-makers. Most of these activities are of a public nature, for the benefit of the community at large and individual households. Financing for sanitation mainly originates from two sources: the household and the public sector (Evans, 2001). Trying to mobilize individual household financial resources for activities targeted at the broader community has, however, proven difficult. This raises one of the main challenges of developing financing mechanisms for sanitation: How can the needs, interests and finances of individuals and households be effectively coordinated and reconciled with those at the community/national level? Ideally, this should be achieved in a way to recover costs, but also to ensure equitable access to sanitation, particularly for poorer members of society.

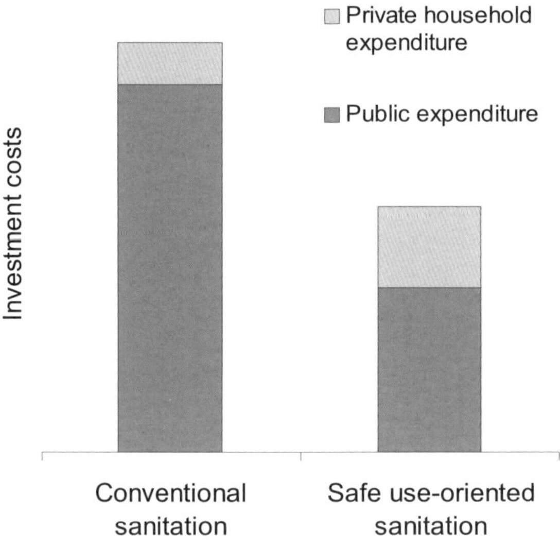

Figure 9.3
The cost structures of conventional and safe use-oriented sanitation systems (Werner et al., 2004)

Sanitation systems that recover excreta and greywater for use in agriculture generally have a different cost structure, and appropriate financing mechanisms may be needed to support private households in their decision to install them. As shown in Figure 9.3, the total costs to install such systems tend to be lower than for more conventional sanitation systems. In comparison with traditional decentralized sanitation (such as pit latrines or VIPs), they normally provide permanent solutions and thus do not have to be replaced when full, representing an incremental saving over an extended period of time. However, although the overall costs are lower, the initial costs to be covered by the private household may be higher as a result of having to replace or transform domestic sanitary facilities (e.g. by installing a urine diversion toilet).

Innovative financing alternatives, including start-up funds, community-based finance programmes, micro-credit programmes or targeted subsidies, which are easily understood by households, may therefore be required. These should put particular emphasis on the possibility of financing the users' investment for on-site and neighbourhood systems. Unlike rural areas, the systems for densely populated urban areas often cannot be left to the individual choice of the households. A common acceptable solution must be found, which may even be stipulated in legislation. Financial mechanisms will also be necessary in such cases to ensure that a uniform system can be adopted. Financing mechanisms should explicitly target the poorest, as they often pay higher costs for services than middle-class families (Mehta & Knapp, 2004). A sensitive use of these mechanisms is essential to ensure that proper support is given with maximum effect.

Experience from projects around the world has shown that subsidized installation of sanitation facilities does not guarantee their proper use and maintenance. Often the opposite is true, and toilets are converted into storerooms, households do not connect to sewers and wastewater treatment plants fail to work properly (Mehta & Knapp, 2004). Subsidies should therefore be focused on assisting households to obtain sanitation facilities that meet their needs, that they will use and whose maintenance they can afford. It is frequently more sustainable to spend financial resources on promotional efforts (including hygiene promotion) than to spend them on subsidies for sanitation hardware (WSSCC, 2005).

Households may be willing to pay up to 3% of household income for improved sanitary services, assuming that the household sees the service as necessary and that it actually does represent an improvement in the current situation (Rogerson, 1996). This expenditure also depends on other factors, such as who controls the household finances, ownership of the property where the family lives and the range of sanitary facilities on offer. Understanding what conditions encourage households to invest in sanitation and designing a range of options that respond to their wants and needs may help mobilize finances at the household level. It is clear from experience that household interest in sanitation is unlikely to be driven by health concerns. Comfort and convenience, prestige, permanence of the structure and, of course, costs are much greater motivating factors in the choice of a sanition system. The additional benefits accruing from the safe use of excreta and greywater have also proven attractive to families engaged in agriculture or horticulture. Adopting a demand-driven approach to sanitation should therefore assist households in choosing the system that they want and can afford.

Distribution of excreta and greywater may be a separate operation from their collection and treatment. Separate charges may be applied to individuals or communities using them. The level of these charges should be agreed at the planning stage. The responsible authorities must decide whether they should cover only the operation and maintenance costs or whether the capital costs of the scheme should be recovered as well. There are trade-offs between the desirability of maximum cost recovery and maintaining incentives for the use of excreta and greywater. Some prior investigation of the willingness and ability to pay is therefore essential in determining not only the level of charges, but also the frequency, timing and means of payment. For instance, in many rural settings, an annual charge payable after the harvest season may be the easiest to collect.

Farmers intent on using excreta and greywater in their agricultural production system may be willing to share in the investment in treatment works that are a prerequisite to obtaining use permits. Their contribution may be in cash or in the form of land for treatment and storage facilities.

The possibilities for private sector participation in sanitation systems that safely recover and use excreta and greywater are considerable (see Boxes 9.2 and 9.3). These range from construction of facilities and providing specific elements for them (e.g. urine-separating toilets) to the logistics of safely collecting, transporting and treating excreta and greywater through to their marketing and use. These market openings can also be stimulated and thus create business opportunities, particularly for small- and medium-sized enterprises.

Municipalities may also be able to operate profitable service providers for the management and treatment of faecal sludge in urban centres (see Boxes 9.2 and 9.3).

Box 9.2 Private sector providers of sanitation services

Factors influencing emptying service delivery for pit latrines and septic tanks

When the pits of on-site sanitation systems are full, they are emptied by cesspit trucks or manually. The financial, institutional and regulatory framework determines largely where and how the faecal sludges are deposited. To reduce cost, the truck drivers in many places sell the sludge to local farmers or dump the product on open spaces or into the drainage systems at the shortest possible distance.

Private cesspit emptying companies are often not legally recognized by the local authorities, even though they may constitute the only initiative catering for faecal sludge collection and disposal. In most cases, a fee structure and money flow procedures have become established without any legal control, resulting in emptying fees affordable to only a few and in indiscriminate dumping of faecal sludge. Experiences in the field show that the emptying service is cost-effective. Proper regulatory mechanisms, private sector competition and the development of economic incentives could help ensure that the collected sludge is delivered to a designated treatment site.

Faecal sludge emptying and haulage: a private sector "stewardship" business

Where the business opportunity exists, the faecal sludge emptying and haulage service is dominated by small-scale private entrepreneurs owning one or a few cesspit trucks. They often hold a share of >70% of this business, in spite of the lack of legal status. Table 9.1 highlights the importance of small-scale sanitation stewardship entrepreneurs, with examples from Ghana, Nepal, Senegal and Viet Nam, respectively, and illustrates the profit potential for faecal sludge removal services. The potential for strengthening the roles of private entrepreneurs in the safe management of faecal sludge exists. The policy framework should facilitate their role in providing safe services.

Table 9.1 Importance of small-scale private sanitation stewardship in faecal sludge management

	Kumasi	Dakar	Hanoi City	Kathmandu
Population (millions)	1.5	2.1	1.5	0.8
Share of population on on-site sanitation	60	60	90	–
Share of installations emptied mechanically (%)	90	70	90	64
Number of cesspit trucks in operation	25	± 100	40	8
Share of private business (%)	80	75	66	70
Total volume of faecal sludge hauled per day (m^3)	200–300	550	300–400	30–50
Average emptying cost per trip (€)	30–40	30–40	20–30	16–22
Yearly turnover/truck (k€)	30–60	20–30	10–20	10–15

Source: Data compiled from a field survey by Department of Water and Sanitation in Developing Countries (SANDEC) and its partners (Centre Régional pour l'eau Potable et l'Assainissement a faible coût (CREPA), Burkina Faso, Center for Environmental Engineering for Towns and Industrial Areas (CEETIA), Viet Nam, Environment and Public Health Organization (ENPHO), Nepal); prepared by Doulaye Koné and Martin Strauss, SANDEC / Swiss Federal Institute for Environmental Science and Technology (EAWAG); Strauss et al., 2003.

Box 9.3 Innovative money flows for improved faecal sludge management

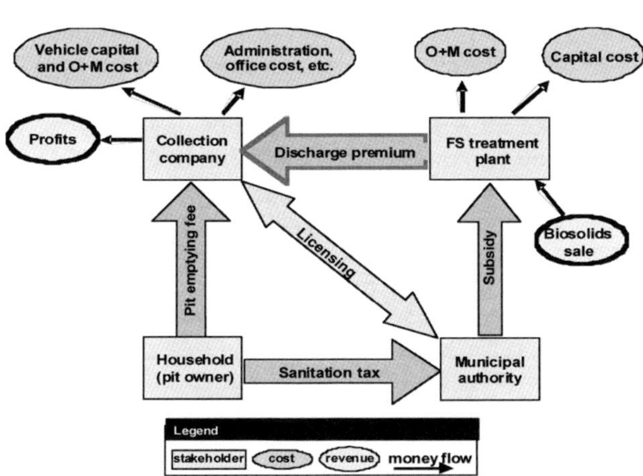

Figure 9.4
Scheme of innovative money flows in faecal sludge management
(O+M = operation and maintenance; FS = faecal sludge)

Sustainable environmental sanitation may be achieved or enhanced only by applying appropriate financial incentives and sanctions (Wright, 1997). Hence, municipalities must devise an effective sanctioning system (e.g. by imposing fines or non-renewal of faecal sludge collection contracts with entrepreneurs) and an incentive-based policy by, among others, paying entrepreneurs for delivering faecal sludge to the legally designated treatment or disposal site.

The potential business opportunity is shown in Figure 9.4. It is based on a rigorous economic analysis of the business opportunities and potential of existing and expected future key players. It analyses conditions under which each player can make a profit, based on their operation and maintenance costs, capital costs, margins of profit and potential for improving the service delivery. The development of the money flow model presented in Figure 9.4 implies a participatory consultation with key stakeholders (households, entrepreneurs, authority representatives, technical services, farmers, etc.). Hence, the project development process should be guided by a thorough stakeholder analysis study and stakeholder involvement process study.

Figure 9.4 illustrates such a financial scheme, the most crucial element of which is the payment to collectors for faecal sludge brought to the treatment site (discharge premiums). The flux reversal principle is about to be introduced in the city of Danang, Viet Nam. The city of Ouagadougou, Burkina Faso, is planning to pay collectors the equivalent of €3.70 per standard truck load on delivery of faecal sludge to the new wastewater/faecal sludge treatment scheme to reduce illegal and illicit dumping of faecal sludge or use of untreated faecal sludge in agriculture. For faecal sludge management to function on a sustainable basis, national or municipal governments must consider providing subsidies, recoverable partly by a tax on water, wastewater or sanitation charged to households. The rationale for such a policy is to render pit emptying affordable to all urban dwellers, to enable entrepreneurs to operate faecal sludge services with adequate profit margins and to keep prices for biosolids usable in agriculture competitive. Intensive information, awareness raising and social/commercial marketing campaigns are needed to render new money flow procedures acceptable to the urban customers and to induce the demand of farmers for biosolids.

Sources: Wright (1997); CREPA-Senegal (2002); Strauss et al. (2003).

9.3 Market feasibility

In planning for greywater and excreta use, it is important that the market feasibility be assessed. Market feasibility may refer to the ability to sell (treated) greywater and excreta to producers, or it can refer to the marketability of agricultural products grown with the use of excreta and greywater (see Table 9.2). For selling treated greywater and excreta, it is important to have an idea of how much people are willing and able to pay. Assessing the marketability is particularly important when crop restriction in agriculture is being considered as a partial health protection measure. Producers should be consulted as to which crops can be restricted. If farmers or market gardeners cannot make a suitable return on their products, then produce or waste application restrictions are likely to fail. Equally, if the excreta are to be used for gas or energy generation, it should also be ascertained if this could be achieved at a competitive price compared with that of other sources of energy.

Table 9.2 Market feasibility: planning questions

Product for sale	Key questions
Greywater and excreta	- What is the price for the treated greywater and excreta that people are willing and able to pay?
	- What is the demand in the project area for treated greywater and excreta?
	- Are there extra costs required to get the treated greywater and excreta to where it will be used (e.g. pumping costs, transport, etc.)?
Produce	- Are products (e.g. plants, biogas) acceptable to consumers?
	- Can producers earn acceptable returns with restricted application and produce?
	- Is the project capable of supplying products that meet market quality criteria (e.g. microbial standards for products to be exported)?

Any agricultural product grown with the use of treated greywater and excreta must be acceptable to the consumers. If the public perception of these products is negative, even if the quality meets WHO or national performance criteria, then farmers still may be unable to sell their produce. If agricultural products require post-harvesting processing, the cost and availability of these services need to be considered. In some cases, it will be necessary to actively market products to increase demand and profit potential. Currently, however, the management and use of most treated excreta and greywater are decentralized, often at household level, and they are used in subsistence rather than commercial agriculture and horticulture.

10
POLICY ASPECTS

The safe management and use of excreta and greywater in agriculture are facilitated by the appropriate policies, legislation, institutional framework and regulation at the international, national and local levels. In many countries, these frameworks are lacking or are insufficiently developed. This chapter looks at different policy and institutional aspects that will help promote the safe use of excreta and greywater. It also gives some country-specific policy/legal/regulatory examples. A policy framework should be based on a holistic approach that maximizes the public health protection and environmental benefits from the point of excreta and greywater generation through application to final product consumption.

Policy is the overall framework that sets national development priorities. It can be influenced by international policy decisions, by international treaties or commitments or by the policies of multilateral development institutions. Policy leads to the creation of relevant legislation. Legislation establishes the responsibilities and rights of different stakeholders. The institutional framework determines which agency has the lead responsibility for creating regulations (often as part of a consultative process) and who has the authority to implement and enforce the regulations (Figure 10.1).

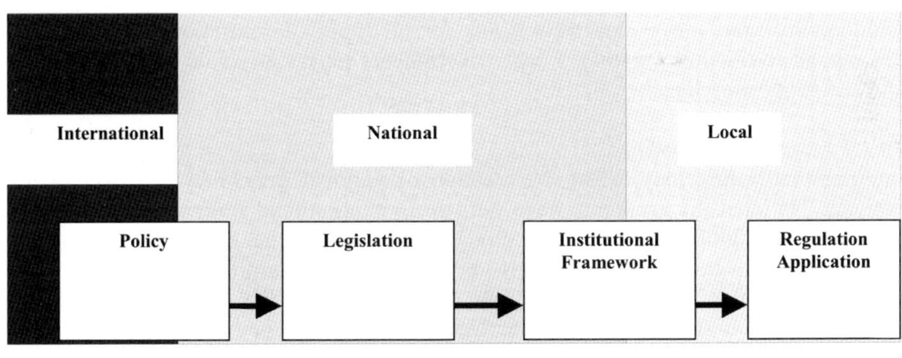

Figure 10.1
Policy framework

10.1 Policy

Policy is the set of procedures, rules and allocation mechanisms that provide the basis for programmes and services. Policies set priorities, and associated strategies allocate resources for their implementation. Policies are implemented through four types of policy instruments (Elledge, 2003):

1) *Laws and regulations:* Laws generally provide the overall framework. Regulations provide the more detailed guidance and may be developed at the national, regional or local level by different authorities as set out in legislation. Regulations are rules or governmental orders designed to control or govern behaviour and often have the force of law. Regulations for excreta and greywater use can cover a wide range of topics, including the practices of service providers, design standards, tariffs, treatment requirements, health-based targets and monitoring requirements, crop restrictions, environmental protection and contracts. These regulations, especially treatment and operational monitoring, have to be appropriate to local conditions.
2) *Economic measures:* Examples of economic measures are user charges, subsidies, incentives and fines. User charges, or tariffs, are charges that households and enterprises pay in exchange for the removal of human excreta

and greywater. Subsidies are allocations in cash or kind to communities and households for establishing recommended types of sanitation facilities or services and for the use of excreta and greywater in agriculture. Fines are monetary charges imposed on enterprises and people for unsafe disposal, emissions and/or risky hygienic behaviours and practices, which are a danger to people and the environment.

3) *Information and education programmes:* These programmes include public awareness campaigns and educational programmes designed to generate demand and public support for efforts to expand sanitation and hygiene services and encourage the safe use of excreta and greywater in agriculture.
4) *Assignment of rights and responsibilities for providing services:* National governments are responsible for determining the roles of national agencies and the appropriate roles of the public, private and non-profit sectors in programme development, implementation and service delivery.

The legislation resulting from policies for the safe use of excreta and greywater should establish a clear functional framework of how the sanitary system should operate. It should be directed explicitly at the correct level (household, district, municipality) and make clear provisions for all types of sanitation systems (from centralized to on-site systems). Local governments play a key role in implementing and enforcing such legislation.

10.1.1 International policy

International policy may affect the creation of national greywater and excreta use policies. National governments have numerous international obligations. They may originate from global treaties and conventions (such as the Basel, Rotterdam and Stockholm conventions). They may be linked to commitments made in the international arena (e.g. the Millennium Development Goals, or recommendations from the Commission on Sustainable Development). Or they may result from the conditions negotiated for loans and credits from international development banks and agencies. National policies for the safe use of excreta and greywater in agriculture will have to be in harmony with this international framework.

Another major issue is the international trade in food products. Those that are raised in compliance with the WHO *Guidelines for the safe use of wastewater, excreta and greywater* are internationally recognized as being developed within an appropriate risk management framework. This can help to facilitate international trade in agricultural products grown with the use of wastewater, excreta and greywater.

10.1.2 National greywater and excreta use policies

Policy priorities for each country are necessarily different to reflect local conditions. National policy on the use of excreta and greywater in agriculture needs to consider the following issues:

- health implications of excreta and greywater use in agriculture;
- requirements for a health impact assessment at the planning stage of proposed projects;
- water scarcity;
- wetland, coastal zone and biodiversity conservation;
- resource recovery and recycling;
- resource availability;
- sociocultural factors that influence practices and acceptability of excreta and greywater use;

- capacity to effectively treat excreta and greywater;
- capability and capacity to implement health protection measures to safely manage excreta and greywater use;
- impacts if excreta and greywater are not used in agriculture;
- impacts on household nutrition, food security and local economy;
- numbers of people dependent on excreta and/or greywater use in agriculture for their livelihoods;
- trade implications of growing crops with the use of treated excreta and/or greywater.

Responsibility for excreta and greywater use is often poorly anchored in existing policy and institutional structures. It may be divided arbitrarily between institutions working in public health, water resources management, agriculture and rural development or between town municipalities and regional and national governments. This may result in uncoordinated approaches and strategies, without an overall institutional responsibility. As most of the excreta and greywater management issues are likely to occur at the household or community level, policies should be clearly based on a local approach. Policies developed for sanitation also apply to the safe use of excreta and greywater and are best enforced by local governments and authorities.

In addition to public health aspects, environmental concerns are important in developing excreta and greywater use policies. National policies can strive to reduce environmental damage by requiring appropriate treatment chains and may also encourage the beneficial recycling of water and nutrient resources. This is apparent in relation to phosphorus, an important nutrient in excreta and greywater and indispensable in agriculture for crop development, but also a major cause of eutrophication if it ends up in freshwater bodies.

10.1.3 Greywater and excreta in integrated water resources management

In many arid and semi-arid countries, the renewable freshwater resources available are already heavily exploited. Integrated water resources management, as defined by the Global Water Partnership (GWP, 2000) is a process that promotes the coordinated development and management of water, land and related resources, in order to maximize the resultant economic and social welfare in an equitable manner without compromising the sustainability of vital ecosystems.

Increasingly, the management of excreta and greywater is considered in the broad framework of integrated water resources management. Greywater may represent a reliable water source with constant flows even in the dry season, and excreta a constant source of organic material, nutrients and energy. Their productive use should figure prominently in water resources management, as it enables communities to reserve and preserve higher-quality water resources (i.e. uncontaminated groundwater or surface water), as well as to improve soil structure and fertility. Excreta and greywater use policies emphasize approaches that reduce environmental contamination and promote safe resource use. Of equal importance at the policy level is the fact that commercial fertilizers may not be an option for many farmers, due to high costs. Plant nutrients present in excreta and greywater are readily available, and their use helps to reduce reliance on commercial fertilizers for crop production.

10.2 Legislation

Legislation may facilitate technical incentives and financing mechanisms. In addition, legislation defines responsibilities and cooperation between relevant stakeholders, including the private sector, and appropriates financial resources for capacity building and training and for monitoring, implementation and maintenance. It provides a basis for enforcement of consistent standards for excreta and greywater collection, treatment and use to be complied with by other sectors (e.g. education, housing construction, workplace safety, etc.). Effective laws and regulations establish both incentives for complying and sanctions for not complying with the requirements (WHO, 2004a).

Often it may be sufficient to amend existing laws, but sometimes new legislation is required. The following areas deserve attention:

- define institutional responsibilities or allocate new powers to existing bodies;
- establish roles and relationships between national and local government levels;
- create rights of access to and ownership of greywater and excreta, including public regulation of its use;
- establish land tenure;
- develop public health and agricultural legislation concerning greywater and excreta quality standards, produce restrictions, application methods, occupational health, food hygiene and other preventive measures linked to health-based targets as deemed relevant.

An example of legal provisions conducive to the recycling of wastewater, excreta and greywater comes from Sweden and is presented in Box 10.1.

10.2.1 Institutional roles and responsibilities

Legislation may be required to establish a national coordinating body for excreta and greywater use and to set up local bodies to manage individual schemes. These will require a certain degree of autonomy from central government and the ability either to charge for the excreta and greywater they distribute or to sell any agricultural produce. Working within an existing institutional framework may be preferable to creating a new one.

At a national level, the safe use of excreta and greywater in agriculture is an activity that touches the responsibilities of several ministries or agencies. Normally, the development of policies to encourage the safe use of excreta and greywater would involve a consultative process between different agencies/institutions with overlapping responsibilities. Examples of ministries, authorities or agencies that have jurisdiction over the use of greywater and excreta in agriculture may include:

- *Ministry of Agriculture:* overall project planning; management of state-owned land; installation, operation and maintenance of irrigation infrastructure; agricultural research and extension, including training; control of product marketing.
- *Ministry of Environment:* sets excreta and greywater treatment and effluent quality standards based on environmental concerns, establishes practices for protecting water resources (both surface water and groundwater) and the environment; establishes monitoring and analytical testing protocols; manages and validates the environmental impact assessment process.
- *Ministry of Health:* health protection, particularly establishment of health-based targets (for treated excreta and greywater, products; health protection measures), monitoring procedures and methods and schedules for treated excreta and greywater; health education; disease surveillance and treatment; manages and validates the health impact assessment process.

- *Ministry of Water Resources:* incorporation of excreta and greywater use into integrated water resources planning and management.
- *Ministry of Energy:* integration of energy generation by the anaerobic treatment of excreta and greywater into national energy plans.
- *Ministry of Education:* develop school curricula concerning sanitation and personal and domestic hygiene and safe practices related to the use of excreta and greywater.
- *Ministry of Public Works/Local Government:* excreta and greywater collection, treatment and use.
- *Ministry of Finance and Economic Planning:* economic and financial appraisal of projects; import control; development of financing mechanisms for excreta and greywater conveyance and treatment and use infrastructure.

Box 10.1 Legislation: promoting or preventing?

The Swedish Environmental Code contains an example of legislation where the use and saving of resources are in focus. The objective states:

The purpose of this Code is to promote sustainable development, which will assure a healthy and sound environment for present and future generations....

The Environmental Code shall be applied in such a way as to ensure that: [...] 5. Reuse and recycling, as well as other management of materials, raw materials and energy are encouraged with a view to establishing and maintaining natural cycles. [...]

This aim is underlined in Chapter 2 of the Code, which states:

Persons who pursue an activity or take a measure shall conserve raw materials and energy and reuse and recycle them wherever possible. Reference shall be given to renewable energy sources.

This article ensures that the aim of conserving raw materials and resources is as important as the aim of minimizing emissions of pollutants, etc. Recycling of nutrients is now stipulated in the provisions, for example, for small wastewater plants for single-family houses.

Other ministries and government agencies, for example those concerned with land tenure, rural development, cooperatives and women's affairs, may also be involved.

Cooperation between the relevant agencies will require effective communications between the technical staff involved. Some countries, especially those facing water scarcity, may find it advantageous to establish an executive body, such as an interagency technical standing committee, under the aegis of a lead ministry (Agriculture or Water Resources) or possibly a separate organization (with both government and private funding sources), to be responsible for the development, planning and management of excreta and greywater use projects. Professionals involved in this will be required to develop skills in intersectoral negotiation and decision-making.

In many countries, the establishment of an ad hoc committee may be sufficient. Alternatively, existing organizations may be given responsibility for this intersectoral issue, or parts of it: for example, a National Water Board may be given responsibility for the safe use of wastewater, excreta and greywater in aquaculture/agriculture/energy generation. Such an organization should have the power to convene a committee of representatives from the different agencies with relevant responsibilities, which, in turn, will provide the interagency or interministerial mechanism to inform others of the challenges/opportunities in developing safe approaches in this connection.

For example, in Uganda, an Inter-Ministerial Steering Committee was set up as a policy- and strategy-making body to oversee activities related to water supply, sanitation and hygiene. It was made up of the permanent secretaries and directors from the ministries of Health, Water, Lands and Environment, Gender, Labour and Social Development, Local Government, Education and Sports, Finance Planning and Economic Development. The role of this committee was to review the overall water supply, sanitation and hygiene policy, coordinate and promote convergence between sectoral activities and promote appropriate changes in policies for sectoral programmes and projects.

In countries with a federal administration with a higher or lower degree of decentralization, such arrangements for interagency collaboration will be important at the appropriate levels. Whereas the general framework of greywater and excreta use policy and standards may be defined at the national level, the regional body will have to interpret and adapt these for effective implementation under local conditions.

Individuals collecting greywater and excreta and managing a scheme will often be under municipal control. If greywater and excreta use is to be promoted in the context of a national policy, this implies careful coordination and definition of the relationship between local and national government. On the one hand, it may be necessary for the national government to offer incentives to local authorities to promote safe use of greywater and excreta; on the other hand, sanctions of some sort may have to be applied to ensure that schemes are implemented without significant risk to public health.

Local governments usually have the authority to develop their own regulations within the national legal framework. For example, they should be able to collect fees for greywater and excreta treatment or other services, issue permits, conduct inspections, develop produce restrictions, inspect markets and develop decentralized greywater and excreta treatment and use facilities.

Permits may be issued by the local agriculture or water resources administration or by the body controlling the greywater and excreta distribution system for the use of excreta and greywater from a public conveyance network. Provision of such permits could be made conditional on the correct observance of sanitary practices regarding application methods, produce restriction and exposure control.

It is common for the agencies administering the distribution of greywater and excreta to deal with the landowners through users' associations, which may develop from traditional institutions. Permits to use greywater and excreta can then be issued to the associations, which simplifies the administrative task of dealing separately with a large number of small users. It also delegates to the associations the task of enforcing the regulations that must be complied with for a permit to be renewed.

A joint committee or management board, which may include representatives of these associations, any particularly large users, the authorities that collect and distribute the greywater and excreta, and also the local health authorities, is required. Even in small organizations, some form of arrangement, such as a committee with community representatives, is important for the users to participate in the management of the project. In some cases, farmers will be able to directly negotiate contracts for a specified supply of treated greywater and excreta with the treatment utility.

10.2.2 Other roles and responsibilities

The number of stakeholders that may be involved in the safe use of excreta and greywater can be quite large and may include individuals, groups, institutions or organizations with different needs and concerns. A detailed stakeholder analysis is normally carried out at the start of activities to identify those that will be of relevance and how large stakeholder groups may be effectively addressed and represented.

The stakeholder analysis given below provides a generic overview of the possible stakeholders in excreta and greywater use programmes:

- *Users of sanitation facilities:* These are most often the individual households. In rural areas, the households are usually the final decision-makers, responsible for the construction and maintenance of the sanitation facilities as well as the collection and treatment of the excreta and greywater; in urban areas, households may be marginally involved, with service providers collecting the excreta and greywater for further secondary off-site treatment, generally against payment. The households can help drive the process forward by adopting good sanitation and hygienic practices, innovating, taking action, talking to the neighbours about solving local problems and encouraging political representatives to support locally developed solutions.
- *Users of the treated excreta and/or greywater:* These may be the users of the sanitation facilities themselves, farmers in nearby areas or, in urban settings, market gardeners or communities involved in (peri-)urban agriculture.
- *Community-based organizations and self-help groups:* These support the households by organizing the delivery of the different services needed (e.g. maintenance of the facilities or the collection and treatment of the final treated products) and the use of the produced fertilizer at the level of the community-based organization or neighbourhood groups.
- *Nongovernmental organizations:* These provide information and raise awareness among potential users. They also often advise the households on the use of sanitation systems and support (poor) households in the contact with, for example, financing institutions and municipalities.
- *Service providers:* Service providers encompass a group of diverse stakeholders engaged in public or private market-oriented activities of service provision. These include planners, consultants, producers/suppliers, construction companies, utility providers and companies involved in excreta and greywater collection, transport and treatment. Farmers also act as service providers by collecting and treating excreta from the users of the sanitation facilities.
- *Developers and investors:* Developers and investors from either the private or public sector may initiate the construction of residential units. The decision of developers and investors to introduce systems for the safe use of excreta and/or greywater is often tightly related to the demand for the treated product. They are often actively involved in the planning and implementation process of an entire programme.
- *Financial institutions:* The introduction of new infrastructure generally requires that the investment and operation costs be secured.
- *Research institutions:* These may be universities or other research-oriented institutions or organizations that can provide evidence and advice to programme initiators, developers, municipalities and nongovernmental organizations.

- *International organizations:* International organizations can ensure that external funds for sanitation hardware are bundled with appropriate hygiene promotion and sanitation marketing activities; encourage governments to consider appropriate, cheaper and more sustainable sanitation systems; finance local sanitation research; develop guidance and tools for facilitating good practice; disseminate information; actively endorse the idea of flexible technical norms and standards to allow for innovation where excreta and greywater use is promoted; and offer support in adopting the legislative and regulatory framework to facilitate safe use and resource efficiency as part of sanitation systems.

Table 10.1 Different factors influencing stakeholders on the adoption of safe use systems

Principal stakeholders	Examples of motivating factors	Examples of constraints
I. Users of sanitation facilities: households, neighbourhoods, tourists, pupils, employees.	No odour, hygiene improvement, structural stability, local physical factors (high groundwater table, rocky ground, etc.), reduced costs, increased comfort, improvement of quality of life, greater security (in-house construction), interest in treated products, prestige, ecological reasons, water scarcity, unreliable water supply.	Habits, taboos, hygienic concerns, unfamiliarity, fear of loss of comfort, unavailability of structural elements, legislative restrictions, economic factors (e.g. for start-up, etc.).
II. Users of treated products.	Economic reasons, local and reliable availability of agricultural inputs (water, nutrients, organics), increase of crop yields for either the market or family needs, improvement of self-sufficiency, ecological reasons.	Habits, taboos, lack of logistics, fear of negative consumer perception, fear of negative long-term effects on soil.
III. Community-based organizations and self-help groups.	Failure of conventional/existing sanitation system, local improvement of quality of life, Agenda 21, MDGs, interest in treated products, reduced costs, local physical factors (high groundwater table, rocky ground, etc.).	Habits, taboos, lack of information, insufficient financing, inappropriate legislation, influence of interest groups, hygienic concerns.
IV. Nongovernmental organizations.	Failure of conventional/existing sanitation systems, economic reasons, ecological reasons, agricultural reuse of treated products, improve quality of life, etc.	Habits, taboos, lack of information, insufficient financing, inappropriate legislation, influence of interest groups, hygienic concerns.
V. Local authorities, government institutions.	Political reasons, economic reasons, ecological reasons, Agenda 21, MDGs, failure of conventional/existing sanitation system, possibility of financial support, sustainability of system, support regional self-sufficiency, promotion of (urban) agriculture, job (and income) creation, long-term security of social services (water supply, etc.).	Habits, taboos, lack of information, lack of start-up funds, insufficient financing, monitoring of treatment/ handling, etc., more difficult for decentralized system, distrust of alternative systems, not recognized as state of the art technology, reluctance to change status quo, contradiction of existing legal framework/long-term plans, powerful lobby from conventional centralized sanitation industry, corruption.

Table 10.1 (continued)

Principal stakeholders	Examples of motivating factors	Examples of constraints
VI. Service providers: planners/consultants, builders, maintenance service providers, producers of equipment, providers of collection, treatment, transport and marketing of the treated products.	Increased profit, opening up of a potentially huge new market, request/need for particular product, further develop their own know-how, ethical/ecological reasons.	Absence of technical knowledge, absence of products, inappropriate legislation, lack of suitable tools, economic interest of (waste) water monopolies, fear of failure (economic risk), not yet recognized as state of the art, reluctance to make the necessary increase in effort, lack of experience in decentralized planning/participation, lack of start-up funds, fear of reduced profit margins in smaller/decentralized projects, regulatory obstacles.
VII. Developers and investors.	Increase attractiveness of developments (eco-label), safe and secure "management" (especially in tourist areas), user satisfaction, economic reasons, legal requirements.	Absence of service logistic, habits, taboos, lack of information, lack of start-up funds, monitoring of treatment/handling, etc., more difficult for decentralized system, distrust of alternative systems, not recognized as state of the art technology, reluctance to change status quo, contradiction of existing legal framework / long-term plans, powerful lobby from conventional centralized sanitation industry, corruption, less "commission" for projects.
VIII. Financial institutions.	Economic reasons, failure of existing/conventional systems, improving sustainability, guarantee repayment of credit.	Absence of specific financing instruments, not recognized as state of the art technology, need for research and development.
IX. Research institutions.	Need for research and development, availability of research funds, ecological reasons.	Availability of research funds, prestige.
X. International organizations.	Political reasons, improvement of public health, pro-poor development goals, improvement of livelihood, social/economic/ecological sustainability, Agenda 21, MDGs, failure of conventional/existing sanitation system	Culture, habits, taboos, lack of information, monitoring of treatment/handling more difficult in a de-centralized system, distrust of innovative systems, reluctance to change, contradiction with existing legal framework, powerful lobby of conventional sanitation industry

Source: Adapted from GTZ (2003); UNESCO/GTZ (2006).

Table 10.1 presents some of the factors that may either motivate different stakeholders to adopt or discourage them from adopting safe use systems. A participatory approach is essential where the stakeholders have the possibility to voice their motivations and reservations. Equally important is dealing with the constraints raised. Mapping the motivations and constraints is a useful task, which should be adapted during the course of the project, becoming increasingly specific with time.

10.2.3 Rights of access

Farmers will be reluctant to install infrastructure or treatment facilities unless they have some confidence that they will continue to have access to the greywater and excreta. Permits dependent on efficient or sanitary practices by the farmers may regulate this access. Legislation may therefore be required to define the users' rights of access to the greywater and excreta and the powers of those entitled to allocate or regulate those rights.

10.2.4 Land tenure

Security of access to greywater and excreta is worth little without security of land or water tenure. Existing tenure legislation is likely to be adequate for most eventualities, although it may be necessary to define the ownership of virgin land newly brought under cultivation. If it is decided to amalgamate individual agricultural areas under a single management, powers of compulsory purchase may be needed.

10.2.5 Public health

The area of public health includes rules governing crop restrictions and methods of application, as well as quality standards for treated greywater and excreta, which may require an addition to existing regulations. It may include application requirements or required withholding periods between application and harvest. It also covers other aspects of health protection, such as the promotion of hygiene and other health issues, occupational health and food hygiene, which are unlikely to need any new measures. Consumers also have the right to expect safe products.

Legislation on the use of excreta and greywater, intended for the protection of public health, should be based on the health-based targets and health protection measures discussed in chapters 4 and 5 of this volume of the Guidelines.

10.3 Regulation

Regulations are the rules that specify actions that need to be performed by the users (can be individuals or communities, etc.) of excreta and greywater. Regulations are usually created through a consultative process led by an administrative authority, with a delegated responsibility in legislation. Regulations governing the use of excreta and greywater should be practical and focus on protecting public health (other issues will also be relevant, e.g. environmental protection). Regulations should also establish requirements to obtain permits, specify the risk management approaches that will be required in different settings, describe water quality/produce monitoring requirements, create disease surveillance requirements and develop financing mechanisms. Most importantly, regulations should be feasible to implement under local circumstances. Box 10.2 provides an example of regulations that affect the use of excreta and greywater in South Africa, and Box 10.3, the development of municipal regulations through consultation with various stakeholders in Tepoztlán, Mexico.

A framework of regulations could be set up around the different health protection measures (i.e. excreta and greywater treatment, use restriction, application, exposure

Box 10.2 National Building Regulations in South Africa

The National Building Regulations state that waterborne sewage and chemical closets are the only acceptable indoor toilets. The assumption is that municipalities will automatically be able to treat the sewage and safely discharge it to the environment. The safe use of excreta and greywater could be incorporated into the standards by allowing the choice of different technologies, e.g. different types of toilets or storage and treatment systems that facilitate the safe use of excreta and greywater. The National Building Regulations could allow the use of different systems if, for example, the owner of the building and/or the municipality can demonstrate that they can comply with system operation and treatment requirements.

Box 10.3 Developing a municipal regulation for the city of Tepoztlán in Mexico

The content of a regulatory framework for a municipality with regard to sanitation is being proposed for the municipality of Tepoztlán in Mexico. The regulation will be developed after extensive consultation with key local and national stakeholders and in parallel with proposals for appropriate institutional reforms to ensure their effective application. This municipal regulation will contain the following specifications:

a. Basic principles and rules taking into account particularities of the municipality.
b. Inclusion of rules for construction permits and new urban developments.
c. Policy and procedures regarding water management and sanitation, including assessment and monitoring.
d. Specify concrete measures and actions regarding sanitation that should be undertaken by the municipality.
e. Adapting local regulations to federal and regional legislation to avoid conflicting jurisdictions and to promote concurrent jurisdictions.
f. Institutional mechanisms of participation of the local population in the process of municipal management in specific affairs of importance such as sanitation, with specific emphasis on surveillance.
g. Definition of minimum norms of quality of the public services offered by the municipality.
h. Requirements for housing development to fulfil the regulation in relation to sanitation and other issues.
i. Establishing proper incentive systems for conversion and retrofitting of conventional technology towards alternative sanitation technologies that facilitate the safe use of excreta and greywater.
j. Implementation of registers and inventories of waters and soils.
k. Improving the tariff system collection.

A bottom-up strategy is thus proposed, where appropriate regulation for a municipality, in this case Tepoztlán, could serve as a model for other municipalities and gradually influence regulation at other levels of government.

control). Regulations may already exist for some of the protective measures. Without some complementary measures, such as regulations that control market hygiene (e.g. availability of adequate sanitation and safe water supplies and market inspectors), safe food products grown in compliance with the excreta or greywater regulations could easily become recontaminated in the market, mitigating any impact of previous public health protective measures that have been implemented (see Table 10.2 for examples of activities that might require regulations).

10.4 Development of a national policy framework

In developing a national policy framework for the safe use of excreta and greywater in agriculture, it is important to define the objectives of the policy, assess the current policy environment and develop a national approach.

10.4.1 Defining objectives

The use of greywater and excreta can have one or more of several objectives. Defining these objectives can help to start the planning and implementation process (Mills & Asano, 1998). The main objectives might be:

- to increase national or local economic development;
- to increase crop production;
- to increase energy production;
- to augment freshwater supplies and otherwise take full advantage of the resource value of greywater and excreta;
- to manage greywater and excreta in a cost-effective, environmentally friendly manner;
- to improve household income, food security and/or nutrition.

Where greywater and excreta are already used, sub-objectives might be to incorporate health and environmental safeguards into management strategies or improve produce or yields through better practice.

Table 10.2 Examples of activities that might be covered in regulations

System components	Regulatory considerations
Greywater and excreta	Access rights; tariffs; management (e.g. municipalities; communities, user groups, etc.)
Conveyance	Responsibility for building infrastructure and operations and maintenance, pumping costs, delivery trucks
Treatment	Treatment requirements depending upon final use; process requirements
Monitoring	Types of monitoring (e.g. process monitoring, analytical, parameters), frequency, location, financial responsibilities
Greywater and excreta application	Fencing, need for buffer zones
Produce restrictions	Types of produce permitted, not permitted, enforcement, education of users/public
Exposure control	Access control for use areas (e.g. sign posting, fences), protective clothing requirements, provision of water and sanitation facilities for workers, hygiene education responsibilities
Market hygiene	Market inspection, provision of safe water and adequate sanitation facilities at markets
Financial authority	Mechanisms for charging tariffs, collecting fines
Enforcement	Mechanisms for ensuring regulatory compliance

10.4.2 Analysis of the existing policy framework

The right formal and informal policy framework can facilitate the safe use and management of excreta and greywater. Existing practices, habits and customs need to be integrated to understand what actions should be taken to reduce risks and maximize benefits.

An existing policy framework facilitates, impedes or is neutral towards the safe use of excreta and greywater. The most practical approach is from a "what is not strictly prohibited" rather than from a "what is specifically allowed?" perspective. This analysis should include the whole handling chain, from point of household generation through conveyance, storage, treatment, use and product consumption. Coordination of many authorities/agencies at the community level will be helpful, and the analysis of the existing framework should have that objective in focus.

As legal, institutional, cultural and religious contexts differ, it is not possible to prescribe a specific methodology for institutional analysis that functions globally. The questions in Table 10.3 should be seen as examples for a structured approach with the aim of identifying the system. Is the purpose to use the excreta and greywater at the household level and then to delegate responsibility to individual households? Or is the system to be operated by a municipality? What permits are necessary? Is it possible for local farmers to sell their crops after using these substances? The framework should not be prescribing specific technologies, but it should be based on the principles of maximizing public health and environmental protection and identifying the necessary changes within the existing institutional framework. Once an analysis is completed, it will be helpful to develop an action plan.

Table 10.3 Structured questions providing input for an institutional analysis of excreta and greywater use

Questions regarding…	Examples of relevant questions
…the legal framework	Does the existing legal framework adequately govern excreta and greywater use?
	Are existing regulations appropriate? Or do existing regulations conflict with desired outcomes for the use?
	Are national policies within the sector based on appropriate levels of legality? Are there barriers or obstacles resulting from the legal basis of excreta or greywater use?
	Are these policies sufficiently comprehensive to allow institutions to develop strategies and action plans to act upon them?
	Are these national policies compatible with other relevant national policies and regulations, for example, environment, public health, education and decentralization?
	Are the policies more appropriate for one or more target groups or areas (e.g. urban areas, small towns, rural areas)?
	Do laws or by-laws cover responsibilities of landlords for providing adequate storage or treatment facilities for tenants?
	What challenges and possibilities exist within the spatial planning and building codes? How is construction permitted or restricted?
	What is stated in technical norms and standards?[a]
	To what extent can neighbours have opinions on land use? Do these rights pose challenges?
	Who has the right to use the resource (e.g. water)?
	Will the owner of the resource, such as the land and water, be entitled to compensation?
	What is stated in the health legislation?
	What is stated in the infectious disease protection legislation?
	Are there environmental quality standards regulating effluent quality?
	Are there legislative obstacles hindering the commercialization of products cultivated with human excreta?
	Is authorization or notification needed for different aspects of the recycling scheme?
	Is there legislation that, in practice, suppresses the development of recycling-oriented sanitation systems?
	Who enforces the rules?
	What is the legal status of excreta and greywater? Covered or excluded?
	How is the flow of different fractions regulated (keeping excreta and greywater separate throughout collection/transport/use)?
	Does the existing legal framework direct the excreta and greywater flow towards use or towards deposition/discharge?
	Who has a right of access to excreta and greywater?
	Are quality standards in place for excreta and greywater, restrictions on crop use, application methods, occupational health, food hygiene, etc?

Table 10.3 (continued)

Questions regarding...	Examples of relevant questions
...the relevant authorities	Who has the responsibility to make legislation/regulation on different levels?
	What are the appropriate standards for excreta and greywater use?
	Is there coordination between the relevant authorities in terms of resposnsibility?
	Is there a clear and proper division of powers/finances/competence?
	What supportive policies are there? Is there a coordination of water and sanitation policies with environmental and agricultural policies?
	Are there action plans connected to the policies?
	What are the roles and relationships between national and local governments?
	Do authorities comply with legislation/regulations? Does the national or state-level government intervene when national policies are not implemented?
...the informal institutions	What are the attitudes, human and organizational behaviour, codes of conduct and behavioural patterns from an excreta and greywater use perspective[b]
	Is there compliance with legislation/regulation[c]?
...other issues	Is there a potential for corruption?
	Are there any other competing interests with the excreta and greywater?

[a] Many existing standards (national or municipal) are based on those developed in industrialized countries, under conditions different from those applying in developing countries, and so they are often inappropriate. Part of launching a household-centred environmental sanitation approach should therefore be to secure a moratorium on the application of existing standards to the programme area, and part of the overall exercise should be to try to identify standards that would be more appropriate because they meet the basic purpose of standards, to ensure that everyone has a healthy life (WSSCC, 2005).

[b] It is important to remember that informal institutions are more resilient towards change than formal ones (Hukkinen, 1999).

[c] Many of the problems related to the legal field have to do with a strong dichotomy between legislation and reality. Some countries may have advanced legislation and comprehensive policy and planning instruments, but poor law enforcement and poor implementation of plans and policies. Any effort to build a different legal framework must tackle this issue in order to promote laws that are in accordance with the complexities that the different actors will have to deal with when applying or being affected by the legislation concerned (Johansson & Kvarström, 2005).

Source: Adapted from Elledge et al. (2002).

10.4.3 Development of action plans

Analysis of the existing legal framework may find that new institutions, laws or regulations are warranted or that existing frameworks should be modified to accommodate the safe use of excreta and greywater.[1] New tasks within the changed framework may be included in action plans. Action plans should be output oriented with monitoring mechanisms. Developing an action plan may include consideration of the following elements:

- **Institutional reform action**
  - adding sanitation and resource recycling into poverty reduction strategy papers
  - allocation of new or changed powers to existing bodies

[1] Institutional change is a complex process and depends on (i) the stability characteristics of institutions, (ii) the sources of change, (iii) the agent of change and (iv) the direction of change and path dependence (North, 1990). Institutions typically change incrementally rather than instantaneously, which means that short-term profitable opportunities cumulatively create the long-term path of change (Seppälä, 2002).

- the creation of new authorities or new tasks for old authorities
- development of new policies (see above for key features of sanitation policies)
- coordination of policies
- creation of economic incentives, removal of economic hindrances
- new/changed legislation/regulation[1]
  - e.g. identification of environmental quality standards, identification of time period to respect between excreta/greywater amendment event and harvest
  - One way to keep legislation modern for a longer time period is to make it less detailed and specific. For the sanitation case, one way of achieving this is to avoid mentioning technologies in legislation/ regulation, but rather focus on functions that the sanitation services should provide. A function, or performance or criteria, approach opens up for innovative technologies/systems as long as they comply with the criteria identified in the legislation/regulation.
- action plans to enforce existing/new regulations
  - Better compliance with existing laws and rules and in many cases also reformed legislation are needed, as both these issues are important and intimately related. Better rules may foster different policies and help, among other things, to get better compliance. However, new laws and rules have to be coupled with concrete and specific application and enforcement of the law.
- reallocation of financial resources
- creation of monitoring mechanisms
- creation of financial mechanisms allowing the safe use of excreta and greywater (e.g. microfinance, revolving funds, etc.)
- completed decentralization processes[2]

- **Change in ways of working**
  - continuous stakeholder involvement in order for legislation/regulation and institutions to be viable and accepted by the public
  - enhanced cooperation between existing authorities
  - execution of integrated planning approaches[3]
- **Piloting**
  - If the institutional framework does not embrace the safe use of excreta and greywater, identification of waiver possibilities in order to conduct use in pilot projects may be essential for decision-making. The programmes should be integrated, encompassing sanitation, health and hygiene, nutrient/resource recycling and food security.

---

[1] Legislation/regulations should create conditions that favour innovation (in both technology and financing mechanisms); define cooperation between relevant stakeholders, including the private sector; and allocate financial resources to capacity building, training and monitoring implementation and maintenance (WHO, 2004a).

[2] If you apply the household-centred environmental sanitation approach to planning of urban environmental sanitation services, it is important to decentralize powers and functions, since it builds on both bottom-up and top-down approaches to service provision planning (WSSCC, 2005).

[3] Household-centred environmental sanitation is a multisector, multiactor approach to delivering urban environmental sanitation services, where urban environmental sanitation services comprise not only sanitation but also storm water and solid waste as well as water provision. In this way, the stakeholders have opportunities to participate in the planning, implementation and operation of urban environmental sanitation services, which is believed to increase their sustainability (WSSCC, 2005).

- **Information, education, communication**
  - awareness-raising campaigns at different levels[1]
  - development of local guidelines for the safe use of excreta and greywater in agriculture
  - capacity-building efforts (e.g. bringing together more resources, stronger institutions, better trained people and improving skills; WHO, 2004a)
    - training regulators so that they know how to support, regulate and control systems for the safe use
  - information sharing through conferences, workshops and other forums
  - information and education programmes (see, for example, WHO's sanitation and hygiene promotion programming guide; WHO, 2005b).

10.4.4 Research

Research on minimizing health impacts associated with use of excreta and greywater in agriculture should be conducted at national institutions, universities or other research centres. It is important to conduct research at the national level, because data concerning local conditions are the most important for developing effective health protection measures and may well vary considerably between countries. Pilot schemes can be developed to investigate feasible health protection measures and answer production-related questions. In situations where excreta and greywater use is practised in small-scale diffuse facilities, often at the household level, national research may be used to validate health protection measures and then develop guidelines and standards to be used by small-scale farmers. Research results should be disseminated to various groups of stakeholders in a form that is useful to them.

A pilot project is particularly useful in countries with little or no experience of managing excreta and greywater use in agriculture or when the introduction of new techniques is envisaged. Health protection is an important consideration, but there are other questions that are difficult to answer without local experience of the kind a pilot project can give. These questions are likely to include important technical, social and economic aspects. A pilot scheme can help to identify potential health risks and develop ways to control them.

Pilot projects should be planned — that is, a variety of crops (both old and new) should be investigated, with different application rates. Information is required not only on yields, but also on levels of toxic metals, organic chemicals and pathogens typically present in the region in local waste and their effects on the environment.

A pilot project should be carefully planned so that the work involved is not underestimated and can be carried out correctly; otherwise, repetition is required. After the experimental period, a successful pilot project may be translated into a demonstration project with training facilities for local operators and farmers.

---

[1] The main reason for awareness raising, on a decision-maker level, with regard to the use of excreta and greywater is that the possibilities it entails are relatively unknown. However, extensive, unregulated use of wastewater occurs in many cities today (e.g. Dakar), even if the main reason for farmers to divert raw wastewater to agricultural or horticultural fields might be to capture water rather than nutrients. Awareness-raising campaigns geared towards farmers should thus address the health risks associated with the use of raw wastewater/excreta and highlight the nutrient value of treated excreta. Awareness raising for safe excreta and greywater use applies also to engineers, planners and even sanitation professionals. There is an overall need to broaden the nature of the debate concerning the role of sanitation and the aims of sanitation provision.

11
PLANNING AND IMPLEMENTATION

The safe use of greywater and excreta in agriculture requires adopting an appropriate planning approach at both the national level and the individual project level, with health as a first priority. Planning strategies, including communication with different groups of stakeholders, have been dealt with in chapter 10. The present chapter describes other planning and implementation issues, partly adapted to the local level.

11.1 Adopting an appropriate planning approach

Planning and development of sanitation programmes have been comprehensively addressed elsewhere (see, for example, WSSCC, 2005). This information can be used as a basis for the creation of new programmes. The planning of sanitary systems aimed to use excreta and greywater should take account of certain specific considerations responding to the needs of a safe use-oriented approach:

- *Integrate aspects of safe use in the assessment of the current sanitary situation and in all the planning activities and conceptual work:* When planning systems to safely use excreta and greywater, a broader spectrum of issues has to be considered. These include the assessment of the current agricultural situation, the type of crops cultivated and prevalent agricultural practices. These relate to the water and fertilizer needs, agricultural equipment and irrigation practices. The quality of the irrigation water used relates to the relative risks of contamination as well as livestock production, practices concerning the treatment and use of manure and current and traditional practices of fertilization and soil conservation. Productivity, costs and benefits, farmers' and consumers' perceptions of the use of artificial fertilizer, manure, treated wastewater, greywater and human excreta as well as other aspects should also be considered. In addition to traditional agriculture, excreta and greywater can be and have been applied as fertilizers in areas such as forestry, aquaculture (see Volume 3 of the Guidelines) and market gardening or for energy production.
- *Integrate aspects related to water supply:* As the source separation of excreta and greywater may reduce the amount of treated fresh water used in homes (e.g. to transport excreta in waterborne systems), water supply systems can often be reviewed and modified.
- *Integrate aspects of urban planning:* As excreta and greywater should be used as close to the source as possible to minimize transport requirements, coordination with urban planners may be required (e.g. in order to provide space for the integration of a constructed wetland in an urban park, to support urban agriculture or to provide small-scale service providers with an area for the treatment and storage of excreta in the neighbourhood).
- *Integrate aspects of solid waste management:* The collection, transport, treatment and use of, for example, composted or dehydrated faeces may be carried out as part of a solid waste management programme. In many countries, those responsible for solid waste management have a long experience with organizing the collection and use systems, as well as marketing know-how.
- *Consider a much wider variety of sanitation systems:* A wide array of technical and operational solutions supporting the use of excreta and greywater are available (see chapter 5). Planners may consider a range of different options for the local circumstances. From the users' perspective, the

ability to choose between different effective technology options to fit their household and budgetary needs is vital. Planners should consider the corresponding institutional and management arrangements needed for different excreta and greywater use options.

- *Apply new and wider-ranging decision-making and evaluation criteria for water supply and sanitation services:* Excreta and greywater use systems highlight the widened boundaries of sanitation systems (integrating aspects of agriculture, energy production, nutrition and public health). Traditionally used evaluation criteria (e.g. the limiting parameters for discharge into receiving water bodies) are insufficient to evaluate different sanitation options. Decision-making criteria should support the choice of sustainable systems and include consideration of resource conservation, health impact, economic, environmental and social aspects and the technical functionality of the system.
- *Provide stakeholders with the relevant information, enabling them to make an "informed choice":* The range of possibilities to recover and safely use excreta and greywater is often unknown to most stakeholders (including decision-makers), which limits their ability to make an informed choice of a sanitary system and its components. Suitable information and awareness raising are therefore needed.

In addition, it is valuable to:

- integrate educational, institutional and capacity-building aspects into planning instruments;
- focus on the assessment of the needs of the user of the sanitation, the end users of the treated excreta and greywater and the service providers;
- consider smaller planning units and a greater number of decentralized options.

To successfully integrate the additional considerations of safe use-oriented sanitation systems, an appropriate approach to the planning processes must be adopted. A sound basis for such an approach can be found in the Bellagio Principles (Box 11.1), drawn up by the Environmental Sanitation Working Group of the Water Supply and Sanitation Collaborative Council (WSSCC) and endorsed by the Council during its 5th Global Forum in November 2000 in Iguaçu, Brazil. The principles call for a change of conventional sanitation policies and practices worldwide (WSSCC/EAWAG/SANDEC, 2000).

The WSSCC (WSSCC/EAWAG/SANDEC, 2004) has published an implementation guide for the Bellagio Principles, promoting a household-centred environmental sanitation approach with two main components:

1) The focal point of environmental sanitation planning should be the household, reversing the customary order of centralized top-down planning. The users of the services should have a deciding voice in their design, and sanitation issues should be dealt with as close as possible to the site where they occur. With the household as the key stakeholder, women are provided with a strong voice in the planning process, and the government's role changes from that of provider to that of enabler.
2) A circular system of resource management should be used, emphasizing the conservation, recycling and reuse of resources, in contrast to the current linear sanitation service system.

Box 11.1 The Bellagio Principles

1) Human dignity, quality of life and environmental security at the household level should be at the centre of the new approach, which should be responsive and accountable to needs and demands in the local and national setting;
- Solutions should be tailored to the full spectrum of social, economic, health and environmental concerns;
- The household and community environment should be protected;
- The economic opportunities of waste recovery and use should be harnessed.

2) In line with good governance principles, decision-making should involve participation of all stakeholders, especially the consumers and providers of services;
- Decision-making at all levels should be based on informed choices;
- Incentives for provision and consumption of services and facilities should be consistent with the overall goal and objective;
- Rights of consumer and providers should be balanced by responsibilities to the wider human community and environment.

3) Waste should be considered a resource, and its management should be holistic and form part of integrated water resources, nutrient flow and waste management;
- Inputs should be reduced so as to promote efficiency and water and environmental security;
- Exports of waste should be minimized to promote efficiency and reduce the spread of pollution;
- Wastewater should be recycled and added to the water budget.

4) The domain in which environmental sanitation problems are resolved should be kept to the minimum practical size (household, community, town, district, catchment, city) and wastes diluted as little as possible;
- Waste should be managed as close as possible to the source;
- Water should be minimally used to transport waste;
- Additional technologies for waste sanitization and reuse should be developed.

11.2 Local project planning: specific considerations

Individual project planning requires consideration of different issues, including the involvement of stakeholders through the use of participatory approaches, treatment, crop restriction, waste application, human exposure control, costs, technical aspects, support services and training.

11.2.1 Participatory approaches

Effective sanitation and hygiene programmes need to combine interventions to change behaviour with the selection of the right technology. Changing behaviour requires culturally sensitive and appropriate health education. People need to understand, in terms meaningful to their lifestyles and existing belief systems, why better health depends on the adoption of hygienic practices such as hand washing, the use of sanitation systems for the safe management of excreta and greywater, and safe storage and handling of drinking-water and food. Raising awareness about the importance of sanitation and hygiene may increase motivation to change harmful behaviours. Selecting the right sanitation technology is about having effective alternatives and making the right choice for the specific circumstances.

Making the right choice of technology requires an assessment of the costs (both for building the facility and for operation and maintenance) and its effectiveness in a specific setting. Participatory approaches such as Self-esteem, Associative strengths, Resourcefulness, Action-planning, and Responsibility (SARAR) and its focused application Participatory Hygiene and Sanitation Transformation (PHAST) have been effective in increasing sanitation coverage and good hygiene behaviours. SARAR has

Box 11.2 SARAR programme achievements in Mexico

Since its inception in 2003, the TepozEco Municipal Ecological Sanitation Project has used SARAR participatory tools to involve community groups in deepening their understanding of their environment and to develop strategies for improving water and sanitation services. TepozEco has worked closely with a local youth group in the periurban community of San Juan Tlacotenco. Members of this group have been trained as sanitation promoters and facilitators of the community decision-making process. In San Juan, the SARAR tools have been particularly valuable as a way to explore community perceptions of their problems and needs and to maintain the focus of decision-making within the community itself. For example:

- An adaptation of the extremely versatile *three-pile sorting* activity was used to involve the community in analysing and prioritizing various public services: not surprisingly, water and sanitation were at the top of the list.
- In a subsequent session, the *sanitation ladder* permitted the community to identify and compare the range of basic sanitation technologies available to them and to decide which options would be most appropriate given the particular local context (severe seasonal water shortages; absence of a central sewage system now and for the longer term; moderate to low income; need for inexpensive fertilizer for local crops; and a concern to avoid contamination of local streams at the top of the watershed).
- A *community mapping* exercise, the *story-with-a-gap* and a set of hygiene behaviour *sorting cards* helped the community to identify critical interventions, including greywater and solid waste management.

Sarar Transformación SC, responsible for coordinating the TepozEco, together with El Taller, a partner nongovernmental organization, have produced an Ecological Sanitation Educational Tool Kit, to facilitate the replication of the process in other programmes. The package includes a set of participatory materials as well as illustrated *technical guides* to provide information to the community in a timely and easily assimilated format with the aim to achieve better hygiene and sanitation behaviour as well as make use of accessible fertilizers in a safe way.

Source: Sarar Transformación SC, Mexico, 2005 (R. Sawyer, personal communication)

been used successfully as a core tool to start sanitation programmes in places as diverse as Mongolia, Kyrgyzstan, Mozambique, South Africa and El Salvador. Box 11.2 gives some examples of how SARAR tools have been used within the context of the TepozEco Municipal Ecological Sanitation Project in Tepoztlán, Mexico.

11.2.2 Treatment

The different characteristics of specific treatments available (see chapter 5) allow choices regarding the use of nutrients and soil conditioners from excreta or of water from greywater.

When excreta from many small sources are used, verification monitoring and assessment of the treatment efficiency of all the sources are impossible. Secondary off-site treatment is then an informed choice, especially in cities. The collection, treatment and reuse of the excreta can provide economic incentives to small entrepreneurs. In rural areas, however, farmers who have used raw excreta for years may not be easily persuaded to treat it. This should be dealt with by health educators and extension officers.

Whatever method is used for health protection when using excreta or greywater, its implementation is likely to demand a change in behaviour by a large number of individual users, which needs to be part of a sensitization process. One motivating factor might be the greater convenience and privacy of an in-house toilet, the waste from which can be treated, compared with open defecation.

11.2.3 Crop restriction

Crop restriction is relatively simple to implement where the treated excreta and greywater are used by a small number of large organizations, whether they are private firms, cooperatives, state farms or the municipal authority itself. However, the enforcement of crop restrictions on a large number of smaller farmers can be much more difficult. The products most likely to be excluded, such as vegetables for direct human consumption, are among those that would give higher cash yields than waste use to produce animal feed. Crop restriction is not impossible in such circumstances; it is most likely to succeed where local dietary habits limit the demand for uncooked vegetables and where there are profitable alternative crops for which a market exists.

In some countries, the existing planning structures and procedures allow a firm control of all produce grown, with regular inspection of farms and sanctions against those who deviate from agreed arrangements. Such mechanisms can be used at little extra cost to ensure that produce restrictions are followed.

If there is no local experience of the application of crop restrictions, their feasibility should be tested in a trial area before they are implemented on a wide scale. Such a trial will also give an initial estimate of the resources required for enforcement, as well as clarifying the most suitable institutional arrangements for the implementation of restrictions.

Enforcement may not always be as easy as might at first appear. Although a crop may take months to grow and can be inspected throughout this time, the excreta and greywater may need to be applied for only a few days each month, and this can be concealed, even from vigilant inspectors.

11.2.4 Application

The Agriculture Extension Service or the organization of Farmer Field Schools may be in the best position to promote hygienic practices relating to the application of excreta and greywater in agriculture/horticulture. Where a municipal body controls the source of treated excreta or faecal sludge, it may be able to encourage application before harvest periods by making it available only at certain times of the year. As stated in chapter 4, a withholding time should always apply, in addition to on-site/off-site treatment. Alternatively, the agency controlling distribution of the excreta or greywater may itself assume responsibility for the application of the treated products and charge for this service. The workers handling the excreta would then be the employees of a single entity, which would facilitate exposure control measures among them.

Source separation of urine and faeces may facilitate the application of excreta to a large degree, although if large amounts of nutrients are needed, the urine volume to be transported may prove impractical.

11.2.5 Human exposure control

Measures to reduce exposure to pathogens associated with water and sanitation and to promote good case management are well known components of primary health care. They include health education, particularly regarding domestic hygiene.

An obvious measure is to provide access to safe drinking-water and adequate sanitation. Controlling the exposure of users of excreta may have little effect if they continue to be exposed to infectious agents in their drinking-water and in their domestic environment through lack of these basic facilities. Particular care is required to ensure that the use of excreta or greywater does not cause contamination of nearby wells or other sources of drinking-water.

Where salaried workers are involved, their employers have a responsibility to protect them from exposure to pathogens, which in many countries is set down in existing legislation on occupational health. This may need to be brought to the employers' attention, together with guidance on the measures they should take, such as the issuing of protective clothing, particularly footwear and gloves, although these may not be comfortable in a tropical climate. Any effort to promote the issuing of protective clothing by employers must be accompanied by still greater efforts to convince their employees that they must wear it.

Measures to control the exposure of those who handle the produce can be implemented in much the same way as for farm workers. When produce handlers all work for a small number of employers, exposure control fits into a general programme of occupational health. On the other hand, when a large number of small traders are involved in selling or processing the produce, it will be difficult to implement exposure control measures unless they are all gathered together in a market. Most markets are subject to public health inspection, and basic exposure control measures may be a good thing, whether or not crops produced using wastes are being handled. In addition to protecting produce handlers from contamination, they may help to protect safe produce from becoming contaminated by the handlers. Markets are also good places to advise consumers about the hygienic precautions they should take with the food they purchase.

Residents who are not involved in the use of excreta or greywater are best placed to ensure that their health is not put at risk by those who are, once it has been explained to them what precautions are required and what risks they and their families may run if the precautions are not taken. Of course, a government inspector can ensure that fences are built and warning signs put up, but vigilant neighbours will be the first to notice when they need repair or replacement. The establishment of a residents' health committee can be a focus for a health education campaign, as well as providing a locally controlled institution to monitor the practice of waste use. The treatment and operational guidelines will in most instances safeguard the use.

With respect to intestinal helminth infections, treatment of farm workers, their families and other exposed groups through chemotherapy is relatively easy to administer in a formal programme, although additional health personnel may be required to treat a large population. It can be quite popular and provides an excellent opportunity for follow-up with hygiene education activities to publicize simple measures for personal protection. The employers may pay the cost of chemotherapy where salaried workers or sharecroppers work the fields.

If untreated excreta and greywater are used on many small and scattered fields, there are greater logistic problems. An additional problem arises where the excreta or greywater are used informally or illegally.

11.2.6 Costs

The choice of a sanitation and safe use system should also consider the overall costs — both the initial expense of the technology but also the ongoing costs of operation and maintenance. If the cost of those technologies chosen for implementation is likely to exceed the economic benefit of using the wastes, it is important to consider whether less expensive measures might suffice or whether it is worthwhile to use the wastes at all. In most cases, the benefits are likely to justify the costs, but some financial arrangement is needed to ensure that the costs are met from a suitable source. These aspects have been considered in chapter 8.

11.2.7 Technical aspects

Detailed planning for excreta and greywater use schemes should follow the usual national procedures for project planning, supplemented as necessary by the requirements of external funding agencies and by procedures specific to the nature of the project (excreta and/or greywater use and for the required health protection measures).

All relevant information needs to be collected to allow for decisions on the technical specifications of a new scheme. A checklist of these specifications is presented in Box 11.3.

Box 11.3 Technical information to be included in a project plan

- Current and projected generation rates of the wastes (excreta, sludge or greywater); proportion of industrial effluents; dilution by surface water
- Existing and required waste treatment facilities; pathogen removal efficiencies; physicochemical quality
- Existing and required land areas: size, location and soil types
- Energy requirements and energy potential of excreta/greywater (and possibility to combine with other organic waste)
- Evaporation (need for make-up water)
- Conveyance of treated wastes (collection of treated excreta and sludge by farmers or delivery by treatment authority)
- Storage requirements for the wastes
- Waste application rates and methods
- Types of crops and their requirements for waste quality and supplementary nutrients
- Estimated yields of crops per hectare per year
- Strategy for health protection

For each scheme, the planner should seek to maximize the net annual benefit in a manner consistent with labour constraints and the need to protect health and minimize costs. For this, cost estimates are valuable for the various activities, including major construction works for storage, treatment or transport of wastes, land preparation and necessary infrastructure, and also for staffing, treatment, pumping and maintenance as well as other inputs.

An assessment of the benefits requires a forecast not only of the probable yields of the crops grown but also of their anticipated prices. This, in turn, demands a survey to establish that an adequate market exists for the produce. This is particularly important where produce restriction is to be employed as a health protection measure and where the produce to be grown requires industrial processing; in the latter case, sufficient processing capacity must be available.

Projects for the use of treated excreta and faecal sludge are not static; they take time to be implemented and thereafter to evolve and grow. The plan should allow reasonable time scales for all its aspects: to obtain funding, to execute any necessary construction works and to prepare the ground for the scheme to begin. From then on, it should envisage the configuration of the project in each year of its future existence. For some projects, a long-term planning horizon will be needed.

A modest start is often advisable, followed by a phased expansion of the project in subsequent years. This will allow time to train farmers and staff in new methods and for lessons learnt in the early stages to influence later developments. It will also help to ensure that the level of production does not over-reach the current availability of excreta as fertilizers or the demand for the produce grown.

11.2.8 Support services

Various support services to farmers are particularly relevant to the implementation of health protection measures, and detailed consideration should be given to them at the planning stage in larger schemes. They include the following:

- machinery (sales and servicing, or hire);
- supplementary fertilizers or feed, pumps, nets, protective clothing, etc.;
- extension and training;
- marketing services, especially where new crops are introduced or new land brought into productive use;
- primary health care, possibly including regular health checks for workers and their families.

11.2.9 Training

Training requirements must be carefully evaluated at the planning stage, and often it may be necessary to start training programmes before the project begins.

The likely need for extension services must be assessed and provisions made for them to be available to producers after implementation of the project. Extension officers themselves will need training in the methods appropriate to health protection, as will the staff responsible for enforcing sanitary regulations regarding, among other things, produce restriction, occupational health and food hygiene.

Such training requirements are best met by local technical colleges and universities, but many countries may lack the specific expertise needed; overseas training may then be the only alternative in the short term until sufficient in-country experience is developed. This is an area in which cooperation between neighbouring countries can be especially fruitful.

REFERENCES

Åkerhielm H, Richert Stintzing A (2004). Anaerobically digested source separated food waste as a fertiliser in cereal production. In: *FAO international conference proceedings 2004*. Network on Recycling of Agricultural, Municipal and Industrial Residues in Agriculture (RAMIRAN).

Albrechtsen H-J (1998). *Water consumption in residences. Microbiological investigations of rain water and greywater reuse systems*. Copenhagen, Miljöstyrelsen och Boligministeriet (ISBN 87-985613-9-1).

Anders W (1952). Worm infestation of school children in Berlin. *Gesundheitsdienst*, 14(2):285–286.

Arfaa F, Ghadirian E (1977). Epidemiology and mass treatment of ascariasis in six rural communities in central Iran. *American Journal of Tropical Medicine and Hygiene*, 26:866–871.

Armon R et al. (1994). Residual contamination of crops irrigated with effluent of different qualities: a field study. *Water Science and Technology*, 30(9):239–248.

Armon R et al. (2002). Surface and subsurface irrigation with effluents of different qualities and presence of *Cryptosporidium* oocysts in soil and on crops. *Water Science and Technology*, 46(3):115–122.

Arnbjerg-Nielsen K et al. (2004). *Risikovurdering af anvendelse af lokalt opsamlet fæces i private havebrug*. Project Report to Miljöstyrelsen, Copenhagen.

Asano T, Levine AD (1996). Wastewater reclamation, recycling and reuse: past, present and future. *Water Science and Technology*, 33(10–11):1–14.

Asano T et al. (1992). Evaluation of the California wastewater reclamation criteria using enteric virus monitoring data. *Water Science and Technology*, 26(7–8):1513–1524.

Ashbolt NJ et al. (2006). Microbial risk assessment tool to aid in the selection of sustainable urban water systems. In: Beck MB, Speers A, eds. *Second IWA leading-edge conference on sustainability in water-limited environments*. London, IWA Publishing.

Austin A (2001). Health aspects of ecological sanitation. In: *Proceedings of the 1st international conference on ecological sanitation, Nanning, China, 5–8 November*, pp. 104-111 (http://www.ias.unu.edu/proceedings/icibs/ecosan/austin.html).

Ayers R, Westcott D (1985). *Water quality for agriculture*. Rome, Food and Agriculture Organization of the United Nations (FAO Agriculture and Drainage Paper 29).

Badawy AS, Rose JB, Gerba CP (1990). Comparative survival of enteric viruses and coliphage on sewage irrigated grass. *Journal of Environmental Science and Health, Part A, Toxic/Hazardous Substances and Environmental Engineering*, 25(8):937–952.

Bartram J, Fewtrell L, Stenström T-A (2001). Harmonised assessment of risk and risk management for water-related infectious disease: an overview. In: Fewtrell L, Bartram J, eds. *Water quality: Guidelines, standards and health — Assessment of risk and risk management for water-related infectious disease*. London, IWA Publishing on behalf of the World Health Organization, pp. 1–16.

Bastos RKX, Mara DD (1995). The bacteriological quality of salad crops drip and furrow irrigated with waste stabilization pond effluent: an evaluation of the WHO guidelines. *Water Science and Technology*, 31(12):425–430.

Båth B (2003). [*Field trials using human urine as fertiliser to leeks.*] Uppsala, Department of Ecology and Plant Production Science, Swedish University of

Bentz RR et al. (1975). The incidence of urine cultures positive for *Mycobacterium tuberculosis* in a general tuberculosis patient population. *American Review of Respiratory Diseases*, 111(5):647–650.

Bertaglial M et al. (2005). *Economic and environmental analysis of domestic water systems: a comparison of centralised and on-site options for the Walloon region, Belgium*(http://216.239.59.104/search?q=cache:WXAeDga4KFgJ:www.mariecurie.org/swap).

Beuchat LR (1998). *Surface decontamination of fruits and vegetables eaten raw: a review*. Geneva, World Health Organization (Report No. WHO/FSF/FOS/98.2).

Blum D, Feachem RG (1985). *Health aspects of nightsoil and sludge use in agriculture and aquaculture. Part III. An epidemiological perspective*. Zurich, International Reference Centre for Waste Disposal (IRCWD Report No. 05/85).

Blumenthal U, Peasey A (2002). *Critical review of epidemiological evidence of the health effects of wastewater and excreta use in agriculture*. Unpublished document prepared for the World Health Organization by London School of Hygiene and Tropical Medicine, London (available upon request from WHO, Geneva).

Blumenthal UJ et al. (2000). *Guidelines for wastewater reuse in agriculture and aquaculture: recommended revisions based on new research evidence*. London, Water and Environmental Health at London and Loughborough (WELL Study, Task No. 68 Part 1).

Blumenthal UJ et al. (2001). The risk of enteric infections associated with wastewater reuse: the effect of season and degree of storage of wastewater. *Transactions of the Royal Society of Tropical Medicine and Hygiene*, 95:1–7.

Blumenthal UJ et al. (2003). *Risk of enteric infections through consumption of vegetables with contaminated river water*. London, London School of Hygiene and Tropical Medicine.

Bofill-Mas S, Pina S, Girones R (2000). Documenting the epidemic patterns of polyomaviruses in human populations by studying their presence in urban sewage. *Applied and Environmental Microbiology*, 6(1):238–245.

Brackett RE (1987). Antimicrobial effect of chlorine on *Listeria monocytogenes*. *Journal of Food Protection*, 50:999–1003.

Brandes M (1978). Characteristics of effluents from grey and black water septic tanks. *Journal of the Water Pollution Control Federation*, 50(11):2547–2559.

Cairncross S (1992). *Sanitation and water supply: Practical lessons from the decade*. Washington, DC, The International Bank for Reconstruction and Development/The World Bank (Water and Sanitation Discussion Paper Series, DP No. 9; http://www.wsp.org/publications/LessonsfromtheDecade.pdf).

Cardone R, Fonseca C (2003). *Financing and cost recovery*. Delft, IRC International Water and Sanitation Centre (Thematic Overview Paper) (http://www.irc.nl/page/113).

Carlander A, Westrell T (1999). *A microbiological and sociological evaluation of urine-diverting double-vault latrines in Cam Dum, Vietnam*. Uppsala, Swedish University of Agricultural Sciences (Report No. 44).

Carr R, Bartram J (2004). The Stockholm Framework for guidelines for microbial contaminants in drinking-water. In: Cotruvo J et al., eds. *Waterborne zoonoses: Identification, causes, and control*. London, IWA Publishing, on behalf of the World Health Organization.

Carrique-Mas J et al. (2003). A Norwalk-like virus waterborne community outbreak in a Swedish village during peak holiday season. *Epidemiology and Infection*, 131(1):737–744.

Casanova L, Gerba C, Karpiscak M. (2001). Chemical and microbiological characterization of graywater. *Journal of Environmental Science and Health*, 36(4):395–401.

CDC (2003). *Leptospirosis.* Atlanta, GA, United States Department of Health and Human Services, Centers for Disease Control and Prevention (http://www.cdc.gov/ncidod/dbmd/diseaseinfo/leptospirosis_t.htm).

Chien BT et al. (2001). Biological study on retention time of microorganisms in faecal material in urine-diverting eco-san latrines in Vietnam. In: *Proceedings of the 1st international conference on ecological sanitation, Nanning, China, 5–8 November 2001*, pp. 120–124 (http://www.ias.unu.edu/proceedings/icibs/ecosan/bui.html).

Chorus I, Bartram J, eds. (1999). *Toxic cyanobacteria in water.* Geneva, World Health Organization.

Christova-Boal D, Eden RE, McFarlane S (1996). An investigation into greywater reuse for urban residential properties. *Desalination*, 106(1–3):391–397.

Cifuentes E (1998). The epidemiology of enteric infections in agricultural communities exposed to wastewater irrigation: perspectives for risk control. *International Journal of Environmental Health Research*, 8:203–213.

Cogan TA, Bloomfield SF, Humphrey TJ (1999). The effectiveness of hygiene procedures for prevention of cross-contamination from chicken carcasses in the domestic kitchen. *Letters in Applied Microbiology*, 29:354–358.

Colley DG (1996). Widespread foodborne cyclosporiasis outbreaks present major challenges. *Emerging Infectious Diseases*, 9(4):426–431.

Collins CH, Grange JM (1987). Zoonotic implication of *Mycobacterium bovis* infection. *Irish Veterinary Journal*, 41:363–366.

Cordy G et al. (2003). Persistence of pharmaceuticals, pathogens, and other organic wastewater contaminants when wastewater is used for ground-water recharge. In: *Proceedings of the 3rd international conference on pharmaceuticals and endocrine disrupting chemicals in water, Minneapolis, Minnesota, 19–21 March.* Sponsored by the National Groundwater Association, Westerville, OH.

Cotte L et al. (1999). Waterborne outbreaks of intestinal microsporidiosis in persons with and without human immunodeficiency virus infection. *Journal of Infectious Diseases*, 180:2003–2008.

CREPA-Senegal (2002). *État des lieux de la gestion des boues de vidanges au Sénégal, rapport d'études.* Dakar, Centre Régional pour l'eau Potable et l'Assainissement a faible coût, 174 pp.

Crites R, Tchobanoglous G (1998). *Small and decentralized wastewater management systems*. Boston, MA, McGraw-Hill.

Curtis TP, Mara DD, Silva SA (1992). Influence of pH, oxygen and humic substances on ability of sunlight to damage fecal coliforms in waste stabilization pond water. *Applied and Environmental Microbiology*, 58(4):1335–1345.

Curtis V, Kanki B (1998) *Happy, healthy and hygienic. Vol. 3. Motivating behaviour change*. New York, UNICEF (WES Technical Guidelines Series No. 5).

Cutter SL (1993). *Living with risk: the geography of technological hazards*. London, Edward Arnold Ltd.

Dailloux M et al. (1999). Water and nontuberculosis mycobacteria. *Water Research*, 33(10):2219–2228.

Del Porto D, Steinfeld C (2000). *The composting toilet system book,* version 1.2 updated. Concord, MA, Center for Ecological Pollution Prevention, 235 pp.

Department of Health (2002). *Draft guidelines for the reuse of greywater in Western Australia*. Prepared by the Department of Health, Government of Western Australia, in consultation with the Water Corporation and the Department of Environment, Water and Catchment Protection (http://www.health.wa.gov.au/publications/documents/HP8122%20Greywater%20Reuse%20Draft%20Guidelines.pdf).

Dixon A, Butler D, Fewkes A (1999). Water saving potentials of domestic water reuse systems using greywater and rainwater in combination. *Water Science and Technology*, 39(5):25–32.

Doller PC et al. (2002). Cyclosporiasis outbreak in Germany associated with the consumption of salad. *Emerging Infectious Diseases*, 8(9):992–994.

Dowd SE et al. (2000). Bioaerosol transport modeling and risk assessment in relation to biosolid placement. *Journal of Environmental Quality*, 29(1):343–348.

Drakatos P et al. (2002). Antagonistic action of Fe and Mn in Mediterranean-type plants irrigated with wastewater effluents following biological treatment. *International Journal of Environmental Studies*, 59(1):125–132.

Drangert J (2004a). Requirements on sanitation systems — the flush toilet sets the standard for ecosan options. In: Werner C et al., eds. *Ecosan — Closing the loop. Proceedings of the 2nd international symposium on ecological sanitation, incorporating the 1st IWA specialist group conference on sustainable sanitation, 7–11 April 2003, Lübeck, Germany*. Eschborn, Deutsche Gesellschaft für Technische Zusammenarbeit (GTZ), pp. 117–124.

Drangert J (2004b). *Norms and attitudes towards ecosan and other sanitation systems*. Stockholm, Stockholm Environment Institute (EcoSanRes Publication Series, Report 2004-5).

Drangert J (2006). *Ecological sanitation, urban agriculture and gender in periurban settlements. A comparative multidisciplinary study in Kampala, Uganda, and Kimberley, South Africa*. Stockholm, Sida Department for Research Cooperation (SAREC) / Swedish International Development Cooperation Agency (Sida) (Research Report).

Drewes JE, Heberer T, Reddersen K (2002). Fate of pharmaceuticals during indirect potable reuse. *Water Science and Technology*, 46(3):73–80.

EC (2000). *Working document on sludge*, 3rd draft. Brussels, European Communities.

Echavarria M et al. (1998). PCR method for detection of adenovirus in urine of healthy and human immunodeficiency virus-infected individuals. *Journal of Clinical Microbiology*, 36(11):3323–3326.

EcoSanRes (2005a). *Closing the loop on phosphorus*. Stockholm, Stockholm Environment Institute (EcoSanRes Fact Sheet 4).

EcoSanRes (2005b). *China-Sweden Erdos Eco-town Project, Dong Sheng, Inner Mongolia, China* (http://www.ecosanres.org/asia.htm).

Edwards P (1992). *Reuse of human wastes in aquaculture: A technical review*. Washington, DC, United Nations Development Programme, World Bank Water and Sanitation Program.

Elledge MF (2003). *Thematic overview paper: Sanitation policies*. Delft, IRC International Water and Sanitation Centre (http://www.irc.nl/page/3271).

Elledge MF et al. (2002). *Guidelines for the assessment of national sanitation policies*. Washington, DC, United States Agency for International Development, Environmental Health Project (Strategic Report 2; http://www.schoolsanitation.org/Resources/Readings/SRSanPolFinal.pdf).

Eller G, Norin E, Stenström TA (1996). Aerobic thermophilic treatment of blackwater mixed with organic waste and liquid manure. Persistence of selected pathogens and indicator organisms. *Environmental Research Forum*, 5–6:355–358.

Eriksson E et al. (2002). Characteristics of grey wastewater. *Urban Water*, 4:85–104.

Esrey S (2001). Towards a recycling society: ecological sanitation — closing the loop to food security. *Water Science and Technology*, 43(4):177–187.

Esrey S et al. (1998). *Ecological sanitation.* Stockholm, Swedish International Development Cooperation Agency.

EU Reach Programme (2005). *REACH (Registration, Evaluation and Authorisation of Chemicals)*. Brussels, European Commission (http://europa.eu.int/comm/environment/chemicals/reach.htm).

Evans B (2001). *Financing and cost recovery.* Sanitation Connection, An Environmental Sanitation Network (http://www.sanicon.net/titles/topicintro.php3?topicId=13).

Fane SA, Ashbolt NJ, White SB (2002). Decentralised urban water reuse: the implications of system scale for cost and pathogen risk. *Water Science and Technology*, 46(6–7):281–288.

FAO (1998). *The state of food and agriculture.* Rome, Food and Agriculture Organization of the United Nations.

Faruqui NI, Biswas AK, Bino MJ, eds. (2001). *Water management in Islam.* Ottawa, Ontario, International Development Research Centre/United Nations University Press.

Fattal B et al. (1986). Health risks associated with wastewater irrigation: An epidemiological study. *American Journal of Public Health*, 76(8):977–979.

Feachem RG et al. (1983). *Sanitation and disease — Health aspects of excreta and wastewater management.* Chichester, John Wiley and Sons.

Fernandez RG et al. (2004). Septage treatment using WSP. In: *Proceedings of the 9th international IWA specialist group conference on wetlands systems for water pollution control and the 6th international IWA specialist group conference on waste stabilization ponds, Avignon, France, 27 September – 1 October* (http://www.sandec.ch/FaecalSludge/Documents/Septage%20treatment%20in%20 WSP.pdf).

Fewtrell L, Bartram J, eds. (2001). *Water quality: Guidelines, standards and health — Assessment of risk and risk management for water-related infectious disease.* London, IWA Publishing on behalf of the World Health Organization.

Foster S et al. (2004). *Urban wastewater as groundwater recharge evaluating and managing the risks and benefits.* Washington, DC, The World Bank (Briefing Note 12).

Franceys R, Pickford J, Reed R (1992). *A guide to the development of on-site sanitation.* Geneva, World Health Organization.

Franzén H, Skott F (1999). *A study of the use and functioning of urine-diverting dry toilets in Cuernevaca, Mexico — Virus survival, user attitudes and behaviours.* Uppsala, Swedish University of Agricultural Sciences, International Office (Report No. 85).

Fraústo da Silva JJR, Williams RJP (1997). *The biological chemistry of the elements — The inorganic chemistry of life*. Oxford, Oxford University Press.

Frost JA et al. (1995). An outbreak of *Shigella sonnei* infection associated with consumption of iceberg lettuce. *Emerging Infectious Diseases*, 1:26–29.

Gantzer C et al. (2001). Monitoring of bacterial and parasitological contamination during various treatment of sludge. *Water Research*, 35(16):3763–3770.

Gao XZ et al. (2002). [*Practical manure handbook.*] Beijing, Chinese Agriculture Publishing House (in Chinese).

Geldreich EE (1978). Bacterial populations and indicator concepts in feces, sewage, stormwater and solid wastes. In: Berg G, ed. *Indicators of viruses in waters*. Ann Arbor, MI, Ann Arbor Science Publishers.

Gerba CP et al. (1995). Water quality study of greywater treatment system. *Water Resources Bulletin*, 31(1):109–116.

Gerba CP et al. (1996) Waterborne rotavirus: a risk assessment. *Water Research*, 30(12):2929–2940.

Gittinger JP (1982). *Economic analysis of agricultural projects*. Baltimore, MD, Johns Hopkins University Press.

Graham DY et al. (1994). Norwalk virus infection of volunteers: new insight based on improved assays. *Journal of Infectious Diseases*, 170(1):34–43.

Grange JM, Yates MD (1992). Survey of mycobacteria isolated from urine and the genitourinary tract in south-east England from 1980 to 1989. *British Journal of Urology*, 69:640–646.

Grimason AM et al. (1993). Occurrence and removal of *Cryptosporidium* spp oocysts and *Giardia* spp cysts in Kenyan waste stabilization ponds. *Water Science and Technology*, 27(3–4):97–104.

GTZ (2003). *An ecosan resource book for the preparation and implementation of ecological sanitation projects*. Eschborn, Deutsche Gesellschaft für Technische Zusammenarbeit (GTZ) (http://www.gtz.de/de/dokumente/en-ecosan-source-book-2005.pdfr).

Gunther F (2000). Wastewater treatment by greywater separation: Outline for a biologically based greywater purification plant in Sweden. *Ecological Engineering*, 15:139–146.

Guzha E, Musara C (2004). Assessment of community knowledge, attitudes, practice, behaviour and acceptance of ecological sanitation in peri-urban areas of Harare. In: Werner C et al., eds. *Ecosan — Closing the loop. Proceedings of the 2nd international symposium on ecological sanitation, incorporating the 1st IWA specialist group conference on sustainable sanitation, 7–11 April 2003, Lübeck, Germany*. Eschborn, Deutsche Gesellschaft für Technische Zusammenarbeit (GTZ), pp. 197–202.

GWP (2000). *Integrated water resources management*. Stockholm, Global Water Partnership (Technical Advisory Committee Background Paper No. 4).

Haas CN, Rose JB, Gerba CP (1999). *Quantitative microbial risk assessment*. New York, John Wiley and Sons.

Hamdy EI (1970). Urine as an *Ascaris lumbricoides* ovicide. *Journal of the Egyptian Medical Association*, 53:261–264.

Hanselman TA, Graetz DA, Wilkie AC (2003). Manure-borne estrogens as potential environmental contaminants: a review. *Environmental Science and Technology* 37(24):5471–5478.

Hardy ME (1999). Norwalk and "Norwalk-like viruses" in epidemic gastroenteritis. *Clinics in Laboratory Medicine*, 19(3):675–690.

Harmsen H (1953). Faecal fertilization of vegetables as a health risk for intestinal parasitism, the spread of intestinal disease polio, and epidemic hepatitis. *Munchener Medizinische Wochenschrift*, 95:1301 [cited by Kreuz, 1955].

Haug RT (1993). *The practical handbook of compost engineering*. Boca Raton, FL, Lewis Publishers.

Havelaar AH, Melse JM (2003). *Quantifying public health risk in the WHO guidelines for drinking-water quality: a burden of disease approach.* Bilthoven, National Institute for Public Health and the Environment (RIVM).

Havelaar AH, de Wit MAS, van Koningsveld R (2000). Health burden in the Netherlands (1900–1995) due to infections with thermophilic *Campylobacter* species. Bilthoven, National Institute for Public Health and the Environment (RIVM).

Hazeleger WC et al. (1998). Physiological activity of *Campylobacter jejuni* far below the minimal growth temperature. *Applied and Environmental Microbiology*, 64(10):3917–3922.

Heberer T (2002) Occurrence, fate and removal of pharmaceutical residues in the aquatic environment: a review of recent research data. *Toxicology Letters*, 131(1–2):5–17.

Heberer T, Schmidt-Bäumler K, Stan H-J (1998). Occurrence and distribution of organic contaminants in the aquatic system in Berlin. Part I: Drug residues and other polar contaminants in Berlin surface and groundwater. *Acta Hydrochimica et Hydrobiologica*, 26(5):272–278.

Heinss U, Larmie SA, Strauss M (1998). *Solids separation and pond systems for the treatment of faecal sludges in the tropics: Lessons learned and recommendations for preliminary design*, 2nd ed. Duebendorf, Swiss Federal Institute for Environmental Science and Technology (EAWAG) / Department of Water and Sanitation in Developing Countries (SANDEC) (SANDEC Report No. 05/98; http://www.sandec.ch/FaecalSludge/Documents/Solids_sep_and_pond_treatm_98.pdf).

Heistad A, Jenssen P, Frydenlund A (2001). A new combined distribution and pretreatment unit for wastewater soil infiltration systems. Mancl IK, ed. Onsite wastewater treatment. In: *Proceedings of the 9th international conference on individual and small community sewage systems.* St. Joseph, MI, American Society of Agricultural Engineers, pp. 200–206.

Hinrichsen D, Robey B, Upadhyay UD (1998). *Solutions for a water-short world.* Baltimore, MD, Johns Hopkins University, School of Public Health, Population Information Program, September (Population Reports, Series M, No. 14; http://www.infoforhealth.org/pr/m14edsum.shtml).

Höglund C (2001). *Evaluation of microbial health risks associated with the reuse of source-separated human urine* [PhD thesis]. Stockholm, Royal Institute of Technology, Department of Biotechnology (ISBN 91-7283-039-5; http://www.lib.kth.se/Sammanfattningar/hoglund010223.pdf).

Höglund CE, Stenström TA (1999). Survival of *Cryptosporidium parvum* oocysts in source separated human urine. *Canadian Journal of Microbiology*, 45(9):740–746.

Höglund C, Ashbolt N, Stenström TA (2002). Microbial risk assessment of source-separated urine used in agriculture. *Waste Management & Research: the Journal of the International Solid Wastes and Public Cleansing Association (ISWA)*, 20:150–161.

Holden R, Terreblanche R, Muller M (2004). Factors which have influenced the acceptance of ecosan in South Africa and development of a marketing strategy. In: Werner C et al., eds. *Ecosan — Closing the loop. Proceedings of the 2nd international symposium on ecological sanitation, incorporating the 1st IWA specialist group conference on sustainable sanitation, 7–11 April 2003, Lübeck, Germany*. Eschborn, Deutsche Gesellschaft für Technische Zusammenarbeit (GTZ), pp. 167–174.

Huitema H (1969). The eradication of bovine tuberculosis in cattle in the Netherlands and the significance of man as a source of infection for cattle. *Selected Papers of the Royal Netherlands Tuberculosis Association*, 12:62–67.

Hukkinen J (1999). *Institutions of environmental management: constructing mental models and sustainability*. Routledge/EUI Environmental Policy Series.

Humphries DL et al. (1997). The use of human faeces as fertilizer is associated with increased intensity of hookworm infection in Vietnamese women. *Transactions of the Royal Society of Tropical Medicine and Hygiene*, 91:518–520.

Hutton G, Haller L (2004). *Evaluation of the costs and benefits of water and sanitation improvements at the global level*. Geneva, World Health Organization.

Ijaz MK et al. (1994). Studies on the survival of aerosolised bovine rotavirus (UK) and a murine rotavirus. *Comparative Immunology, Microbiology and Infectious Diseases*, 17(2):91–98.

Ingallinella AM et al. (2002). The challenge of faecal sludge management in urban areas — strategies, regulations and treatment options. *Water Science and Technology*, 46(10):285–294.

Ishikawa T. (1998). Nightsoil in Edo: Ingenious recycling of human waste. *Rivers and Japan*, No. 13, October. Tokyo, Ministry of Construction.

Jawetz E, Melnick JL, Adelberg EA (1987). *Review of medical microbiology*, 17th ed. East Norwalk, CT, Appleton & Lange.

Jenkins MB, Bowman DD, Ghiorse WC (1998). Inactivation of *Cryptosporidium parvum* oocysts by ammonia. *Applied and Environmental Microbiology*, 64(2):784–788.

Jenkins MB et al. (2002). *Cryptosporidium parvum* oocyst inactivation in three soil types at various temperatures and water potentials. *Soil Biology and Biochemistry*, 34(8):1101–1109.

Jenssen PD (2001). Design and performance of ecological sanitation systems. In: *Proceedings of the 1st international conference on ecological sanitation, Nanning, China, 5–8 November 2001*, pp. 120–124 (http://www.ias.unu.edu/proceedings/icibs/ecosan/jenssen.html).

Jenssen PD, Siegrist RL (1990). Technology assessment of wastewater treatment by soil infiltration systems. *Water Science and Technology*, 22(3/4):83–92.

Jenssen PD, Siegrist RL (1991). Integrated loading rate determinations for wastewater infiltration systems sizing. On-site wastewater treatment. In: *Proceedings of the 6th symposium on individual and small community sewage systems, 16–17 December 1991, Chicago, IL*. St. Joseph, MI, American Society of Agricultural Engineers, pp. 182–191 (ASAE Publication 10-91).

Proceedings of the 2nd international symposium on ecological sanitation, incorporating the 1st IWA specialist group conference on sustainable sanitation, 7–11 April 2003, Lübeck, Germany. Eschborn, Deutsche Gesellschaft für Technische Zusammenarbeit (GTZ), pp. 875–881.

Jenssen PD et al. (2004). *Ecological sanitation and reuse of wastewater (ecosan) — a thinkpiece on ecological sanitation*. Report to the Norwegian Ministry of Environment. 18 pp.

Jenssen PD et al. (2005). An urban ecological sanitation pilot study in humid tropical climate. In: *Proceedings of the 3rd international ecological sanitation conference, Durban, South Africa, 23–27 May 2005*. EcoSanRes, pp. 257–265 (http://conference2005.ecosan.org/papers_presented.html).

Jeppesen B (1996). Domestic greywater re-use: Australia's challenge for the future. *Desalination*, 106(1–3):311–315.

Jeppesen B (1996). Domestic greywater re-use: Australia's challenge for the future. *Desalination*, 106(1–3):311–315.

Johansson M et al. (2001). *Urine separation — closing the nutrient cycle.* Stockholm, Stockholm Water Company (http://www.stockholmvatten.se/pdf_arkiv/english/Urinsep_eng.pdf).

Johansson M, Kvarnström E (2005). *A review of sanitation regulatory frameworks.* Stockholm, Stockholm Environment Institute (EcoSanRes Publication Series 2005-1).

Jönsson H, Vinnerås B (2004). Adapting the nutrient content of urine and faeces in different countries using FAO and Swedish data. In: Werner C et al., eds. *Ecosan — Closing the loop. Proceedings of the 2nd international symposium on ecological sanitation, incorporating the 1st IWA specialist group conference on sustainable sanitation, 7–11 April 2003, Lübeck, Germany.* Eschborn, Deutsche Gesellschaft für Technische Zusammenarbeit (GTZ), pp. 623–626.

Jönsson H et al. (1999). [Source separation of urine.] *Wasser & Boden*, 51(11):21–25 (in German).

Jönsson H et al. (2000). [*Recycling source separated human urine.*] Stockholm, Swedish Municipalities Sewage Research Program (VA-FORSK) / VAV (VA-FORSK Report 2000•1) (in Swedish with English summary).

Jönsson H et al. (2005). Ecosan both economical and eco-sane. *Water*, 21 (International Water Association's monthly magazine), June, p. 15.

Kapperud G et al. (1995). Outbreak of *Shigella sonnei* infection traced to imported iceberg lettuce. *Journal of Clinical Microbiology*, 33(3):609–614.

Katzenelson E, Buium I, Shuval HI (1976). Risk of communicable disease infection associated with wastewater irrigation in agricultural settlements. *Science*, 194:944–946.

Kay D et al. (1994). Predicting likelihood of gastroenteritis from sea bathing: results from randomised exposure. *Lancet*, 344(4927):905–909.

Kincaid D, Solomon K, Oliphant J (1996). Drop size distributions for irrigation sprinklers. *Transactions of the ASAE*, 39(3):839–845.

Kirchmann H, Petterson S (1995). Human urine — chemical composition and fertilizer efficiency. *Fertilizer Research*, 40:149–154.

Kitamura T et al. (1994). Transmission of the human polyomavirus JC virus occurs both within the family and outside the family. *Journal of Clinical Microbiology*, 32(10):2359–2363.

Knutsson M, Kidd-Ljunggren K (2000). Urine from chronic hepatitis B virus carriers: Implications for infectivity. *Journal of Medical Virology*, 60(1):17–20.

Kochar V (1979). *Culture–parasite relationship: socio-behavioural regulations of hookworm transmission in a rural West Bengal region.* Varanasi, Banaras Hindu University (Studies in Medical Social Science, No. 1).

Kolsky P, Diop O (2004). *Frameworks for upscaling sustainable sanitation: Issues, principles and experience.* Presentation given at Sustainable Sanitation Seminar, Stockholm Water Week, 15 August 2004.

Koné D, Strauss M (2004). Low cost options for treating faecal sludges (FS) in developing countries — challenges and performance. In: *Proceedings of the 9th international IWA specialist group conference on wetlands systems for water pollution control and the 6th international IWA specialist group conference on waste stabilization ponds, Avignon, France, 27 September – 1 October* (http://www.sandec.ch/FaecalSludge/Documents/FS_treatment_Avignon_2004.pdf).

Koné D et al. (2004). Efficiency of helminth eggs removal in dewaterered faecal sludge by co-composting. In: *People-centred approaches to water and environmental sanitation, Proceedings of the 30th WEDC international conference, Vientiane, Lao People's Democratic Republic, 25–29 October 2004.* Leicestershire, Loughborough University, Water, Engineering and Development Centre.

Koottatep T et al. (2004). Treatment of septage in constructed wetlands in tropical climate — Lessons learnt after seven years of operation. In: *Proceedings of the 9th international IWA specialist group conference on wetlands systems for water pollution control and the 6th international IWA specialist group conference on waste stabilization ponds, Avignon, France, 27 September – 1 October* (http://www.sandec.ch/FaecalSludge/Documents/Paper_7years%20experience%20revised.pdf).

Kosek M, Bern C, Guerrant RL (2003). The global burden of diarrhoeal disease, as estimated from studies published between 1992 and 2000. *Bulletin of the World Health Organization*, 81(3):197–204.

Kowal NE (1985). *Health effects of land application of municipal sludge*. Research Triangle Park, NC, United States Environmental Protection Agency, Health Effects Research Laboratory (Publication No. EPA/600/1-85/015) [cited in USEPA (1999). *Environmental regulations and technology — Control of pathogens and vector attraction in sewage sludge*. Cincinnati, OH, United States Environmental Protection Agency (EPA/625/R-92-013).]

Kozai I (1962). Re-estimation of sodium nitrate as an ovicide used in nightsoil. IV. On the field trial with Na-nitrite-Ca-superphosphate mixture and the effect of its application upon *Ascaris* and hookworm infection among people in treated rural areas of Saitama prefecture. *Japanese Journal of Parasitology*, 11:400–410.

Kreuz A (1955). Hygienic observations on agricultural use of sewage. *Gesundheits-Ingenieur*, 76:206–211.

Kristiansen R, Skaarer N (1979). [Amount and composition of greywater.] *Vann*, 2:151–156 (Official Journal of the Norwegian Water and Wastewater Association) (in Norwegian).

Kunitake T et al. (1995). Parent-to-child transmission is relatively common in the spread of human polyoma JC virus. *Journal of Clinical Microbiology*, 33(6):1448–1451.

Kutsumi H (1969). Epidemiological study of the preventive effect of thiabendazole as an ovicide against human hookworm, *Trichuris* and *Ascaris* infections. *Japanese Journal of Medical Science and Biology*, 22:51–64.

Kvarnström E et al. (2004). Sustainability criteria in sanitation planning. In: *People-centred approaches to water and environmental sanitation, Proceedings of the 30th WEDC international conference, Vientiane, Lao People's Democratic Republic, 25–29 October 2004.* Leicestershire, Loughborough University, Water, Engineering and Development Centre.

Lan Y et al. (2001). Observation on the inactivation effect on eggs of *Ascaris suum* in urine diverting toilets. In: *Proceedings of the 1st international conference on ecological sanitation, Nanning, China, 5–8 November*, p. 125 (http://www.ias.unu.edu/proceedings/icibs/ecosan/yang2.html).

Lang MM, Harris LJ, Beuchat LR (2004). Survival and recovery of *Escherichia coli* O157:H7, *Salmonella*, and *Listeria monocytogenes* on lettuce and parsley as affected by method of inoculation, time between inoculation and analysis, and treatment with chlorinated water. *Journal of Food Protection*, 67:1092–1103.

Larsen PB (1998). [*Allowable pollution loads for contaminated soils.*] Copenhagen, Danish Environmental Protection Agency (Miljöproject 425; ISBN 87-7909-068-0) (in Danish).

Leeming R, Nichols PD, Ashbolt NJ (1998). *Distinguishing sources of faecal pollution in Australian inland and coastal waters using sterol biomarkers and microbial faecal indicators.* Melbourne, Urban Water Research Association of Australia (Report No. 204).

Lemon SM (1997). Type A viral hepatitis: epidemiology, diagnosis and prevention. *Clinical Chemistry*, 43(8 Part 2):1494–1499.

Lens P, Zeeman G, Lettinga G (2001). *Decentralised sanitation and reuse: Concepts, systems and implementation.* London, IWA Publishing, pp. 355–363.

Lentner C, Lentner C, Wink A (1981). *Units of measurement, body fluids, composition of the body, nutrition. Geigy scientific tables.* Basel, Ciba-Geigy.

Li Z et al. (2004). High quality greywater recycling with biological treatment and 2-step membrane filtration. In: Werner C et al., eds. *Ecosan — Closing the loop. Proceedings of the 2nd international symposium on ecological sanitation, incorporating the 1st IWA specialist group conference on sustainable sanitation, 7–11 April 2003, Lübeck, Germany.* Eschborn, Deutsche Gesellschaft für Technische Zusammenarbeit (GTZ), pp. 555–557.

Lindgren S, Grette S (1998). [*Water and sewerage system in Ekoporten, Norrköping.*] Stockholm, SABO Utveckling (Trycksak 13303/1998-06.500) (in Swedish).

Lipton M (1983). *Poverty, under-nutrition and hunger.* Washington, DC, World Bank, World Bank Staff Working Papers.

Mansell J, Drewes J, Rauch T (2004). Removal mechanisms of endocrine disrupting compounds (steroids) during soil aquifer treatment. *Water Science and Technology*, 50(2):229–237.

Manville D et al. (2001). Significance of indicator bacteria in a regionalized wastewater treatment plant and receiving waters. *International Journal of Environmental Pollution*, 15(4):461–466.

Mara DD (1978). *Sewage treatment in hot climates.* Chichester, John Wiley & Sons.

Mara DD (2004). *Domestic wastewater treatment in developing countries.* London, Earthscan Publications.

Mara DD, Silva SA (1986). Removal of intestinal nematode eggs in tropical waste stabilization ponds. *Journal of Tropical Medicine and Hygiene*, 89(2):71–74.

Marschner H (1997). *Mineral nutrition of higher plants*, 2nd ed. London, Academic Press.

Marshall MM et al. (1997). Waterborne protozoan pathogens. *Clinical Microbiology Reviews*, 10(1):67–85.

Matthias A (1996). Atmospheric pollution. In: Pepper IL et al., eds. *Pollution science.* San Diego, CA, Academic Press.

Maxwell D, Levin C, Csete J (1998) *Does urban agriculture help prevent malnutrition: evidence from Kampala.* Washington, DC, International Food Policy and Research Institute, Food Consumption and Nutrition Division (Paper No. 45).

Mead PS et al. (1999). Food related illness in the United States. *Emerging Infectious Diseases*, 5(5):607–625.

Medema GJ, Bahar M, Schets FM (1997). Survival of *Cryptosporidium parvum, Escherichia coli*, faecal enterococci and *Clostridium perfringens* in river water: influence of temperature and autochthonous microorganisms. *Water Science and Technology*, 35(11–12):249–252.

Mehta M, Knapp A (2004). *The challenge of financing sanitation for meeting the Millennium Development Goals.* Washington, DC, Water and Sanitation Programme, African Region, 32 pp. (http://www.wsp.org/publications/af_finsan_mdg.pdf).

Meinhardt PL, Casemore DP, Miller KB (1996). Epidemiologic aspects of human cryptosporidiosis and the role of waterborne transmission. *Epidemiologic Reviews*, 18(2):118–136.

Michel P et al. (2000). Estimation of the underreporting rate for the surveillance of *Escherichia coli* O157:H7 cases in Ontario, Canada. *Epidemiology and Infection*, 125:35–45.

Mills RA, Asano T (1998). Planning and analysis of wastewater reuse projects. In: Asano T, ed. *Wastewater reclamation and reuse.* Lancaster, PA, Technomic Publishing Company, pp. 57–111.

Moe C, Izurieta R (2004). Longitudinal study of double vault urine diverting toilets and solar toilets in El Salvador. In: Werner C et al., eds. *Ecosan — Closing the loop. Proceedings of the 2nd international symposium on ecological sanitation, incorporating the 1st IWA specialist group conference on sustainable sanitation, 7–11 April 2003, Lübeck, Germany.* Eschborn, Deutsche Gesellschaft für Technische Zusammenarbeit (GTZ), pp. 295–302.

Mohr AJ (1991). Development of models to explain the survival of viruses and bacteria in aerosols. In: Hurst CJ, ed. *Modeling the environmental fate of microorganisms.* Washington, DC, American Society for Microbiology, pp. 160–190.

Montangero A, Nguyen T, Belevi H (2004). Material flow analysis as a tool for environmental sanitation planning in Viet Tri, Vietnam. In: *People-centred approaches to water and environmental sanitation, Proceedings of the 30th WEDC international conference, Vientiane, Lao People's Democratic Republic, 25–29 October 2004.* Leicestershire, Loughborough University, Water, Engineering and Development Centre.

Morgan P (2003). *Experiments using urine and humus derived from ecological toilets as a source of nutrients for growing crops.* Paper presented at the 3rd World Water Forum, 16–23 March 2003 (http://aquamor.tripod.com/KYOTO.htm).

Morgan P (2004). *An ecological approach to sanitation in Africa: A compilation of experiences* (EcoSanRes Fact Sheet 12; http://www.ecosanres.org/PDF%20files/Fact_sheets/ESR12lowres.pdf).

Morgan P (2005). *An ecological approach to sanitation in Africa.* Harare, Aquamore.

Morken J (1998). Direct ground injection — a novel method of slurry injection. *Landwards*, winter:4–7.

Mufson MA, Belshe RB (1976). A review of adenovirus in the etiology of acute hemorrhagic cystitis. *Journal of Urology*, 115(2):191–194.

Murray CJL, Acharya AK (1997). Understanding DALYs. *Journal of Health Economics*, 16:703–730.

Murray CJL, Lopez AD, eds. (1996). *The global burden of disease. Vol. 1.* Cambridge, MA, Harvard School of Public Health on behalf of the World Health Organization and the World Bank.

Naturvårdsverket (1995). [*What does household wastewater contain? Nutrients and metals in urine, faeces and dish-, laundry and showerwater.*] Stockholm, Swedish Environmental Protection Agency (Report No. 4425) (in Swedish).

Needham C et al. (1998). Epidemiology of soil-transmitted nematode infections in Ha Nam Province, Vietnam. *Tropical Medicine and International Health*, 3:904–912.

Nolde E (1999). Greywater reuse systems for toilet flushing in multi-storey buildings — over ten years experience in Berlin. *Urban Water*, 1:275–284.

Norin E, Stenström TA, Albihn A (1996). [Stabilisation and disinfection of blackwater and organic waste by liquid composting.] *Vatten*, 52:3 (in Swedish).

North DC (1990). *Institutions, institutional change and economic performance*. Cambridge, Cambridge University Press.

NRMMC, EPHCA (2005). *National guidelines for water recycling: managing health and environmental risks*. Canberra, Natural Resource Management Ministerial Council and Environment Protection and Heritage Council of Australia.

Ollinger-Snyder P, Matthews ME (1996). Food safety: Review and implications for dietitians and dietetic technicians. *Journal of the American Dietetic Association*, 96:163–168, 171.

Olsson Engvall E, Gustavsson O (2001). [Leptospirosis.] In: Källenius G, Svenson SB, eds. [*Zoonoses*.] Lund, Studentlitteratur (in Swedish).

Oragui JI et al. (1987). Removal of excreted bacteria and viruses in deep waste stabilization ponds in northeast Brazil. *Water Science and Technology*, 19:569–573.

Otterpohl R (2002). Options for alternative types of sewerage and treatment systems directed to the overall performance. *Water Science and Technology*, 45(3):149–158.

Ottosson J (2003). *Hygiene aspects of greywater and greywater reuse* [Licenciate thesis]. Stockholm, Royal Institute of Technology, Department of Land and Water Resources Engineering.

Ottosson J, Stenström TA (2003a). Faecal contamination of greywater and associated microbial risks. *Water Research*, 37(3):645–655.

Ottosson J, Stenström TA (2003b). Growth and reduction of microorganisms in sediments collected from a greywater treatment system. *Letters in Applied Microbiology*, 36(3):168–172.

Pahren HR et al. (1979). Health risks associated with land application of municipal sludge. *Journal of the Water Pollution Control Federation*, 51(11):2588–2601.

Palmquist H (2004). *Hazardous substances in wastewater management* [PhD Thesis]. Dr. Scient. Theses 2004:47. Luleå, Luleå University of Technology (ISSN:1402-1544).

Panesar A, Lange J (2001). *Innovative sanitation concept shows way towards sustainable urban development — experiences from the model project "Wohnen & Arbeiten" in Freiburg, Germany* (http://www.gtz.de/ecosan/download/Freiburg-Vauban-Apanesar.pdf).

Peasey A (2000). *Health aspects of dry sanitation with waste reuse*. Loughborough and London, Water and Environmental Health at London and Loughborough, London School of Hygiene and Tropical Medicine, Water, Engineering and Development Centre (WELL Studies in Water and Environmental Health Task No. 324; http://www.lboro.ac.uk/well/resources/well-studies/full-reports-pdf/task0324.pdf).

Pesaro F, Sorg I, Metzler A (1995). *In situ* inactivation of animal viruses and a coliphage in nonaerated liquid and semiliquid animal wastes. *Applied and Environmental Microbiology*, 61(1):92–97.

Petterson SR, Ashbolt NJ (2003). *WHO guidelines for the safe use of wastewater and excreta in agriculture: microbial risk assessment section*. Geneva, World Health Organization (unpublished document, available on request from WHO, Geneva).

Petterson SR, Ashbolt NJ, Sharma A (2001). Microbial risks from wastewater irrigation of salad crops: a screening-level risk assessment. *Water Environment Research*, 72(6):667–672; Errata: *Water Environment Research*, 74(4):411.

Petterson SR, Teunis PFM, Ashbolt NJ (2001). Modeling virus inactivation on salad crops using microbial count data. *Risk Analysis*, 21:1097–1108.

Phi D et al. (2004). *Study on the survival of* Ascaris suum *eggs in faecal matter inside the ecosan toilets built in Dan Phuong – Lam Ha – Lam Dong – Vietnam.* Nha Trang Pasteur Institute, University of Kyoto, NIPPON International Cooperation for Community Development Organisation (NICCO).

Porter A (1938). The larval Trematoda found in certain South African Mollusca with special reference to schistosomiasis (bilharziasis). *Publications of the South African Institute for Medical Research*, 8:1–492 [cited in Feachem et al., 1983].

Prüss A, Havelaar A (2001). The global burden of disease study and applications in water, sanitation, and hygiene. In: Fewtrell L, Bartram J, eds. *Water quality: Guidelines, standards and health — Assessment of risk and risk management for water-related infectious disease.* London, IWA Publishing on behalf of the World Health Organization, pp. 43–59.

Rasmussen G, Jenssen PD, Westlie L (1996). Graywater treatment options. In: Staudenmann J Schönborn A, Etnier C, eds. *Recycling the resource, Proceedings of the 2nd international conference on ecological engineering for wastewater treatment, Waedenswil, Switzerland, 18–22 September 1995*, pp. 215–220 (Environmental Research Forum Vols. 5–6).

Rice AL et al. (2000). Malnutrition as an underlying cause of childhood deaths associated with infectious diseases in developing countries. *Bulletin of the World Health Organization*, 78:1207–1221.

Ridderstolpe P (2004). *Introduction to greywater management.* Stockholm, Stockholm Environment Institute, EcoSanRes (EcoSanRes Publications Series, Report 2004-4; http://www.ecosanres.org/PDF%20files/ESR%20Publications%20 2004/ESR4%20web.pdf).

Robertson LJ, Campbell AT, Smith HV (1992). Survival of *Cryptosporidium parvum* oocysts under various environmental pressures. *Applied and Environmental Microbiology*, 58(11):3494–3500.

Rodhe L, Richert Stintzing A, Steineck S (2004). Ammonia emissions after application of human urine to clay soil for barley growth. *Nutrient Cycling in Agroecosystems*, 68:191–198.

Rogerson CM (1996). Willingness to pay for water: The international debates. *Water SA*, 22(4):373–380.

Romig RR (1990). The effect of temperature and deposition in reservoir sediments or water on the viability of cultured *Giardia intestinalis* cysts, as determined by fluorogenic dyes. *Dissertation Abstracts International Part B – Science and Engineering*, 51(1):82–88.

Rose JB et al. (1991). Microbial quality and persistence of enteric pathogens in graywater from various household sources. *Water Research*, 25(1):37–42.

Roseberry AM, Burmaster DE (1992). Lognormal distribution for water intake by children and adults. *Risk Analysis*, 12(1):99–104.

Rosemarin A (2004). In a fix: The precarious geopolitics of phosphorous. *Down to Earth*, 30 June:27–31 (http://www.sei.se/dload/2004/Rosemarin_NP.pdf).

Samanta BB, van Wijk CA (1998). Criteria for successful sanitation programmes in low income countries. *Health Policy and Planning*, 13(1):78–86.

Schönning C, Leeming R, Stenström TA (2002). Faecal contamination of source-separated human urine based on the content of faecal sterols. *Water Research*, 36(8):1965–1972.

Schönning C et al. (2006). Microbial risk assessment of local handling and use of human faeces. *Journal of Water and Health* (in press).

Seppälä O (2002). Effective water and sanitation policy reform implementation: need for systematic approach and stakeholder participation. *Water Policy*, 4:367–388.

Sharpley AN (1995). Soil phosphorus dynamics: Agronomic and environmental impacts. *Ecological Engineering*, 5:261–279.

Shields AF et al. (1985). Adenovirus infections in patients undergoing bone-marrow transplantation. *New England Journal of Medicine*, 312(9):529–533.

Shrestha RR, Haberl R, Laber J (2001). Constructed wetland technology transfer to Nepal. *Water Science and Technology*, 43(11):345–350.

Shuval HI (1991). Effects of wastewater irrigation of pastures on the health of farm animals and humans. *Revue Scientifique et Technique*, 10(3):847–866.

Shuval HI, Lampert Y, Fattal B (1997). Development of a risk assessment approach for evaluating wastewater reuse standards for agriculture. *Water Science and Technology*, 35(11–12):15–20.

Sidhu J et al. (2001). Role of indigenous microorganisms in suppression of *Salmonella* regrowth in composted biosolids. *Water Research*, 35(4):913–920.

Siegrist RL, Boyle WC (1981). Onsite reclamation of residential greywater, In: *Proceedings of the 3rd national symposium on individual and small community sewage treatment, 14–15 December, Chicago, IL*. St. Joseph, MI, American Society of Agricultural Engineers, pp. 176–186 (Publication 1-82).

Siegrist RL, Tyler EJ, Jenssen PD (2000). *Design and performance of onsite wastewater soil absorption systems*. Prepared for National Research Needs Conference, Risk-Based Decision Making for Onsite Wastewater Treatment, St. Louis, Missouri, 19–20 May 2000. Sponsored by United States Environmental Protection Agency, Electric Power Research Institute's Community

Skjelhaugen OJ (1999). Closed system for local reuse of blackwater and food waste, integrated with agriculture. *Water Science and Technology*, 5:161–168.

Smit J (2000). Urban agriculture and biodiversity. *Urban Agriculture Magazine*, 1(1):11–12.

Smit J, Ratta A, Nasr J (1996). *Urban agriculture, food, jobs, and sustainable cities*. New York, United Nations Development Programme.

Snowdon JA, Cliver DO, Converse JC (1989). Land disposal of mixed human and animal wastes: A review. *Waste Management and Research* 7:121–134.

Solomon EB, Yaron S, Matthews KR (2002). Transmission of *Escherichia coli* O157:H7 from contaminated manure and irrigation water to lettuce plant tissue and its subsequent internalization. *Applied and Environmental Microbiology*, 68(1):397–400.

Squire L, van der Tak HG (1975). *Economic analysis of projects*. Baltimore, MD, Johns Hopkins University Press.

Srikanth R, Naik D (2004). Prevalence of giardiasis due to wastewater reuse for agriculture in the suburbs of Asmara City, Eritrea. *International Journal of Environmental Health Research*, 14(1):43–52.

Stevik TK (1998). *Retention and elimination of pathogenic bacteria percolating through biological filters. Effect of physical, chemical and microbiological factors*. PhD thesis, NLH, Ås, Norway

Stevik TK et al. (1998). Removal of *E. coli* during intermittent filtration of wastewater effluent as affected by dosing rate and media type. *Water Research*, 33(9):2088–2098.

Stevik TK et al. (1999). The influence of physical and chemical factors on the transport of *E. coli* through biological filters for wastewater purification. *Water Research*, 33(18):3701–3706.

Stine SW et al. (2005). Application of microbial risk assessment to the development of standards for enteric pathogens in water used to irrigate fresh produce. *Journal of Food Protection*, 68(5):913–918.

Stott R et al. (1994). *An experimental evaluation of potential risks to human health from parasitic nematodes in wastewaters treated in waste stabilization ponds and used for crop irrigation.* Leeds, University of Leeds, Department of Civil Engineering, Tropical Public Health Engineering (TPHE Research Monograph No. 6).

Strauss M (1985). Health aspects of nightsoil and sludge use in agriculture and aquaculture — Part II: Survival of excreted pathogens in excreta and faecal sludges. *IRCWD News*, 23:4–9. Duebendorf, Swiss Federal Institute for Environmental Science and Technology (EAWAG) / Department of Water and Sanitation in Developing Countries (SANDEC).

Strauss M (1996). Health (pathogen) considerations regarding the use of human waste in aquaculture. In: Staudenmann J, Schönborn A, Etnier C, eds. *Recycling the resource, Proceedings of the 2nd international conference on ecological engineering for wastewater treatment, Waedenswil, Switzerland, 18–22 September 1995*, pp. 83–98 (Environmental Research Forum Vols. 5–6).

Strauss M, Blumenthal UJ (1990). *Human waste in agriculture and aquaculture: utilization practices and health perspectives.* Duebendorf, International Reference Centre for Waste Disposal, 52 pp. (IRCWD Report No. 09/90).

Strauss M et al. (2003). *Urban excreta management — situation, challenges, and promising solutions.* In: Proceedings, Asian Waterqual 2003, IWA Asia-Pacific Regional Conference, Bangkok, Thailand, 20–22 October (http://www.sandec.ch/FaecalSludge/Documents/Urban_Excreta_Management_IWA_Bangkok_03.pdf).

Svensson L (2000). Diagnosis of foodborne viral infections in patients. *International Journal of Food Microbiology*, 59(1–2):117–126.

Tanner R (1995). Excreting, excretors and social policy. Some cross-cultural observations on an underresearched activity. *Journal of Preventive Medicine & Hygiene*, 36 (3/4):1–10.

Tauxe RV, Cohen ML (1995). Epidemiology of diarrheal diseases in developed countries. In: Blaser MJ et al., eds. *Infections of the gastrointestinal tract.* New York, Raven Press, pp. 37–51.

Tessier JL, Davies GA (1999). Giardiasis. *Primary Care Update for Ob/Gyns*, 6(1):8–11.

Teunis PFM et al. (1996). *The dose–response relation in human volunteers for gastro-intestinal pathogens.* Bilthoven, National Institute for Public Health and the Environment (RIVM) (RIVM Report 28450002).

Thomas C, Hill DJ, Mabey M (1999). Evaluation of the effect of temperature and nutrients on the survival of *Campylobacter* spp. in water microcosms. *Journal of Applied Microbiology*, 86(6):1024–1032.

Thorup-Kristensen K (2001). Root growth and soil nitrogen depletion by onion, lettuce, early cabbage and carrot. *Acta Horticulturae*, 563:201–206.

Tidåker P (2003). *Life cycle assessment of grain production using source separated human urine and mineral fertiliser*. Uppsala, Swedish University of Agricultural Sciences Department of Agricultural Engineering (Report 251; http://www.bt.slu.se/lt_old/Rapporter/Ra251/Report251.pdf).

Tiessen H, eds. (1995). *Phosphorus in the global environment — Transfers, cycles and management*. New York, Wiley (SCOPE 54; http://www.icsu-scope.org/downloadpubs/scope54/TOC.htm).

Trujillo S et al. (1998). Potential for greywater recycle and reuse in New Mexico. *New Mexico Journal of Science*, 38:293–313.

UNESCO/GTZ (2006). *Capacity building for ecological sanitation — concepts for ecologically sustainable sanitation in formal and continuing education.* Paris.

United Nations (2002). *Report of the World Summit on Sustainable Development.* New York, United Nations (http://www.johannesburgsummit.org/html/).

United Nations General Assembly (2000). *United Nations Millennium Declaration. Resolution A/RES/55/2.* New York, United Nations (http://www.un.org/millennium/declaration/ares552e.pdf).

United Nations Population Division (2002). *World urbanization prospects: the 2001 revision.* New York, United Nations Department of Economic and Social Affairs, Population Division (http://www.un.org/esa/population/publications/wup2001/2001WUPCover.pdf).

USEPA (2002). *Onsite wastewater treatment systems manual.* Washington, DC, United States Environmental Protection Agency (EPA/625/R-00/008; http://www.epa.gov/owm/septic/pubs/septic_2002_osdm_prelim.pdf).

Van R et al. (1992). Outbreaks of human enteric adenovirus type 40 and 41 in Houston day care centers. *Journal of Pediatrics*, 120(4):516–521.

Vaz da Costa Vargas S, Bastos RKX, Mara DD (1996). *Bacteriological aspects of wastewater irrigation.* Leeds, University of Leeds, Department of Civil Engineering, Tropical Public Health Engineering (TPHE Research Monograph No. 8).

Venugopalan V (1984). Foreword. In: Roy AK et al., eds. *Manual on the design, construction and maintenance of low-cost waterseal latrines in India.* Washington, DC, World Bank (TAG Technical Note No. 10).

Vinnerås B (2002). *Possibilities for sustainable nutrient recycling by faecal separation combined with urine diversion* [PhD Thesis]. Uppsala, Swedish University of Agricultural Sciences, Department of Agricultural Engineering (Agraria 353; http://www2.gtz.de/ecosan/download/vinneras-nutrient-recycling.pdf).

Vinnerås B et al. (2006). The characteristics of household wastewater and biodegradable solid waste — A proposal for new Swedish design values. *Urban Water Journal*, 3(1):3–11.

Wang JQ (1999). Reduction of microorganisms in dry sanitation due to different adsorbents under low temperature conditions. In: *Abstracts from the 9th Stockholm water symposium, 9–12 August, Stockholm.* Stockholm, Stockholm International Water Institute, pp. 396–398.

Ward BK, Irving LG (1987). Virus survival on vegetables spray-irrigated with wastewater. *Water Resources*, 21:57–63.

Warnes S, Keevil CW (2003). *Survival of* Cryptosporidium parvum *in faecal wastes and salad crops.* Carlow, Teagasc Irish Agriculture and Food Development Authority (http://www.teagasc.ie/publications/2003/conferences/cryptosporidiumparvum).

Watanabe T, San D, Omura D (2002). Risk evaluation for pathogenic bacteria and viruses in sewage sludge compost. *Water Science and Technology*, 46(11–12):325–330.

Water Utility Partnership (undated). Defining legal framework. In: *Water and sanitation for all: A practitioners companion*. Abidjan (http://web.mit.edu/urbanupgrading/waterandsanitation/policies/defining-leg-frame.html).

WCED (1987). *Our common future*. Oxford, Oxford University Press on behalf of the World Commission on Environment and Development.

Werner C et al. (2003). *Ecological sanitation: a source book*. Eschborn, Deutsche Gesellschaft für Technische Zusammenarbeit (GTZ) (http://www2.gtz.de/ecosan/download/ecosan-source-book-3rddraft-eng.pdf).

Werner C et al., eds. (2004). *Ecosan — Closing the loop. Proceedings of the 2nd international symposium on ecological sanitation, incorporating the 1st IWA specialist group conference on sustainable sanitation, 7–11 April 2003, Lübeck, Germany*. Eschborn, Deutsche Gesellschaft für Technische Zusammenarbeit (GTZ), 1004 pp. (ISBN 3-00-012791-7).

Westrell T (2004). *Microbial risk assessment and its implications for risk management in urban water systems* [PhD Thesis]. Linköping, Linköping University, Department of Water and Environmental Studies (ISBN 91-85295-98-1; http://www.urbanwater.org/file/dyn/00000m/3000m/3025i/Kappa%20TW.pdf).

Wheeler JG et al. (1999). Study of infectious intestinal disease in England: rates in the community, presenting to general practice, and reporting to national surveillance. *British Medical Journal*, 318:1046–1050.

WHO (1973). *Reuse of effluents: Methods of wastewater treatment and health safeguards. Report of a WHO Meeting of Experts*. Geneva, World Health Organization (Technical Report Series No. 517).

WHO (1989). *Health guidelines for the use of wastewater in agriculture and aquaculture*. Geneva, World Health Organization (Technical Report Series No. 776).

WHO (1995). *Control of foodborne trematode infections*. Geneva, World Health Organization (Technical Report Series 849).

WHO (1996). *Cholera and other epidemic diarrhoeal diseases control*. Geneva, World Health Organization (Fact sheets on environmental sanitation).

WHO (1999). *Food safety issues associated with products from aquaculture: report of a joint FAO/NACA/WHO study group*. Geneva, World Health Organization (WHO Technical Report Series No. 883).

WHO (2000). *Turning the tide of malnutrition: responding to the challenge of the 21st century*. Geneva, World Health Organization (Report No. WHO/NHD/00.7).

WHO (2003a). *Guidelines for safe recreational water environments. Vol. 1. Coastal and fresh waters*. Geneva, World Health Organization.

WHO (2003b). *The world health report 2003 — Shaping the future*. Geneva, World Health Organization.

WHO (2003c). *Typhoid vaccine*. Geneva, World Health Organization (fact sheet: http://www.who.int/vaccines/en/typhoid.shtml).

WHO (2004a). *Guidelines for drinking-water quality*, 3rd ed. Geneva, World Health Organization.

WHO (2004b). *The world health report 2004 — Changing history*. Geneva, World Health Organization.

WHO (2004c). *The sanitation challenge: Turning commitment into reality*. Geneva, World Health Organization.

WHO (2005a). *Guidelines for safe recreational water environments. Vol. 2. Swimming pools and similar environments*. Geneva, World Health Organization.

WHO (2005b). *Sanitation and hygiene promotion: programming guidance*. Geneva, World Health Organization (http://www.who.int/water_sanitation_health/hygiene/sanitpromotionguide/en/).

WHO, UNDP, WSP (1997). *The PHAST Initiative: Participatory Hygiene and Sanitation Transformation. A new approach to working with communities*. Geneva, World Health Organization.

WHO/UNICEF (2004). *Meeting the MDG drinking water and sanitation target: A mid-term assessment of progress*. Geneva, World Health Organization, United Nations Children's Fund.

Wilhelm C (2004). *Grauwasser-recycling in der wohnbebauung in Peking*. GEP Eitorf, Umwelttechnik GmbH (http://www.fbr.de/fachinfos/pdf_grau/Wilhelm.pdf).

Winblad U, Simpson-Hébert M, eds. (2004). *Ecological sanitation*, rev. ed. Stockholm, Stockholm Environmental Institute.

Wirbelauer C, Breslin ED, Guzha E (2003). Lessons learnt on ecosan in Southern Africa — towards closed-loop sanitation. In: Werner C et al., eds. *Ecosan — Closing the loop. Proceedings of the 2nd international symposium on ecological sanitation, incorporating the 1st IWA specialist group conference on sustainable sanitation, 7–11 April 2003, Lübeck, Germany*. Eschborn, Deutsche Gesellschaft für Technische Zusammenarbeit (GTZ), pp. 135–142.

World Food Programme (1995). *World Food Programme mission statement*. Rome, Food and Agriculture Organization of the United Nations.

Wright A (1997). *Toward a strategic sanitation approach: Improving the sustainability of urban sanitation in developing countries*. Washington, DC, The International Bank for Reconstruction and Development and The World Bank.

WSSCC (2005). *Sanitation and hygiene promotion — programming guidance*. Geneva, Water Supply and Sanitation Collaborative Council.

WSSCC/EAWAG/SANDEC (2000). Bellagio Statement: clean, healthy and productive living. A new approach to environmental sanitation. In: *Bellagio Meeting on Sanitation, 1–4 February 2000*. Geneva, Water Supply and Sanitation Collaborative Council (WSSCC), Swiss Federal Institute for Environmental Science and Technology (EAWAG), and Department of Water and Sanitation in Developing Countries (SANDEC).

WSSCC/EAWAG/SANDEC (2004). *Implementing the Bellagio Principles in urban environmental sanitation services*. Geneva, Water Supply and Sanitation Collaborative Council (WSSCC), Swiss Federal Institute for Environmental Science and Technology (EAWAG), and Department of Water and Sanitation in Developing Countries (SANDEC).

Xu L-Q et al. (1995) Soil-transmitted helminthiases: nationwide survey in China. *Bulletin of the World Health Organization*, 73:507–513.

Yates MV, Gerba CP (1998). Microbial considerations in wastewater reclamation and reuse. In: Asano T, ed. *Wastewater reclamation and reuse*. Lancaster, PA, Technomic Publishing Company, pp. 437–488.

Yates MV, Gerba CP, Kelley LM (1985). Virus persistence in groundwater. *Applied and Environmental Microbiology*, 49(4):778–781.

Zhang Y et al. (2003). Biodiesel production from waste cooking oil: 1. Process design and technological assessment. *Bioresources Technology*, 89(1):1–16.

Zhu T (1998). *Phosphorus and nitrogen removal in light-weight aggregate (LWA) constructed wetlands and intermittent filter systems* [PhD Thesis]. Dr. Scient. Theses 1997:16. Aas, The Agricultural University of Norway.

Annex 1
Glossary of terms used in Guidelines

This glossary does not aim to provide precise definitions of technical or scientific terms, but rather to explain in plain language the meaning of terms frequently used in these Guidelines.

Abattoir – Slaughterhouse where animals are killed and processed into food and other products.

Advanced or tertiary treatment – Treatment steps added after the secondary treatment stage to remove specific constituents, such as nutrients, suspended solids, organics, heavy metals or dissolved solids (e.g. salts).

Anaerobic pond – Treatment pond where anaerobic digestion and sedimentation of organic wastes occur; usually the first type of pond in a waste stabilization pond system; requires periodic removal of accumulated sludge formed as a result of sedimentation.

Aquaculture – Raising plants or animals in water (water farming).

Aquifer – A geological area that produces a quantity of water from permeable rock.

Arithmetic mean – The sum of the values of all samples divided by the number of samples; provides the average number per sample.

Biochemical oxygen demand (BOD) – The amount of oxygen that is required to biochemically convert organic matter into inert substances; an indirect measure of the amount of biodegradable organic matter present in the water or wastewater.

Blackwater – Source-separated wastewater from toilets, containing faeces, urine and flushing water (and eventually anal cleansing water in "washing" communities).

Buffer zone – Land that separates wastewater, excreta and/or greywater use areas from public access areas; used to prevent exposures to the public from hazards associated with wastewater, excreta and/or greywater.

Cartage – The process of manually transporting faecal material off site for disposal or treatment.

Coagulation – The clumping together of particles to increase the rate at which sedimentation occurs. Usually triggered by the addition of certain chemicals (e.g. lime, aluminium sulfate, ferric chloride).

Constructed wetlands – Engineered pond or tank-type units to treat faecal sludge or wastewater; consist of a filtering body planted with aquatic emergent plants.

Cost–benefit analysis – An analysis of all the costs of a project and all of the benefits. Projects that provide the most benefits at the least cost are the most desirable.

Cyst – Environmentally resistant infective parasitic life stage (e.g. *Giardia*, *Taenia*).

Cysticercosis – Infection with *Taenia solium* (pig tapeworm) sometimes leads to cysticerci (an infective life stage) encysting in the brain of humans, leading to neurological symptoms such as epilepsy.

Depuration – Transfer of fish to clean water prior to consumption in an attempt to purge their bodies of contamination, potentially including some pathogenic microorganisms.

Diarrhoea – Loose, watery and frequent bowel movements, often associated with an infection.

Disability adjusted life years (DALYs) – Population metric of life years lost to disease due to both morbidity and mortality.

Disease – Symptoms of illness in a host, e.g. diarrhoea, fever, vomiting, blood in urine, etc.

Disinfection – The inactivation of pathogenic organisms using chemicals, radiation, heat or physical separation processes (e.g. membranes).

Drain – A conduit or channel constructed to carry off stormwater runoff, wastewater or other surplus water. Drains can be open ditches or lined, unlined or buried pipes.

Drip irrigation – Irrigation delivery systems that deliver drips of water directly to plants through pipes. Small holes or emitters control the amount of water that is released to the plant. Drip irrigation does not contaminate aboveground plant surfaces.

Dual-media filtration – Filtration technique that uses two types of filter media to remove particulate matter with different chemical and physical properties (e.g. sand, anthracite, diatomaceous earth).

Effluent – Liquid (e.g. treated or untreated wastewater) that flows out of a process or confined space).

Encyst – The development of a protective cyst for the infective stage of different parasites (e.g. helminths such as foodborne trematodes, tapeworms, and some protozoa such as *Giardia*).

Epidemiology – The study of the distribution and determinants of health-related states or events in specified populations, and the application of this study to the control of health problems.

***Escherichia coli* (*E. coli*)** – A bacterium found in the gut, used as an indicator of faecal contamination of water.

Excreta – Faeces and urine (see also faecal sludge, septage and nightsoil).

Exposure – Contact of a chemical, physical or biological agent with the outer boundary of an organism (e.g. through inhalation, ingestion or dermal contact).

Exposure assessment – The estimation (qualitative or quantitative) of the magnitude, frequency, duration, route and extent of exposure to one or more contaminated media.

Facultative pond – Aerobic pond used to degrade organic matter and inactivate pathogens; usually the second type of pond in a waste stabilization pond system.

Faecal sludge – Sludges of variable consistency collected from on-site sanitation systems, such as latrines, non-sewered public toilets, septic tanks and aqua privies. Septage, the faecal sludge collected from septic tanks, is included in this term (see also excreta and nightsoil).

Flocculation – The agglomeration of colloidal and finely divided suspended matter after coagulation by gentle stirring by either mechanical or hydraulic means.

Geometric mean – A measure of central tendency, just like a median. It is different from the traditional mean (which is called the arithmetic mean) because it uses multiplication rather than addition to summarize data values. The geometric mean is a useful summary when changes in the data occur in a relative fashion.

Greywater – Water from the kitchen, bath and/or laundry, which generally does not contain significant concentrations of excreta.

Groundwater – Water contained in rocks or subsoil.

Grow-out pond – Pond used to raise adult fish from fingerlings.

Hazard – A biological, chemical, physical or radiological agent that has the potential to cause harm.

Health-based target – A defined level of health protection for a given exposure. This can be based on a measure of disease, e.g. 10^{-6} DALY per person per year, or the absence of a specific disease related to that exposure.

Health impact assessment – The estimation of the effects of any specific action (plans, policies or programmes) in any given environment on the health of a defined population.

High-growing crops – Crops that grow above the ground and do not normally touch it (e.g. fruit trees).

High-rate treatment processes – Engineered treatment processes characterized by high flow rates and low hydraulic retention times. Usually include a primary treatment step to settle solids followed by a secondary treatment step to biodegrade organic substances.

Hydraulic retention time – Time the wastewater takes to pass through the system.

Hypochlorite – Chemical frequently used for disinfection (sodium or calcium hypochlorite).

Indicator organisms – Microorganisms whose presence is indicative of faecal contamination and possibly of the presence of more harmful microorganisms.

Infection – The entry and development or multiplication of an infectious agent in a host. Infection may or may not lead to disease symptoms (e.g. diarrhoea). Infection can be measured by detecting infectious agents in excreta or colonized areas or through measurement of a host immune response (i.e. the presence of antibodies against the infectious agent).

Intermediate host – The host occupied by juvenile stages of a parasite prior to the definitive host and in which asexual reproduction often occurs (e.g. for foodborne trematodes or schistosomes the intermediate hosts are specific species of snails).

Legislation – Law enacted by a legislative body or the act of making or enacting laws.

Localized irrigation – Irrigation application technologies that apply the water directly to the crop, either through drip irrigation or bubbler irrigation. Generally use less water and result in less crop contamination and reduce human contact with the wastewater.

Log reduction – Organism removal efficiencies: 1 log unit = 90%; 2 log units = 99%; 3 log units = 99.9%; and so on.

Low-growing crops – Crops that grow below, on or near the soil surface (e.g. carrots, lettuce).

Low-rate biological treatment systems – Use biological processes to treat wastewater in large basins, usually earthen ponds. Characterized by long hydraulic retention times. Examples of low-rate biological treatment processes include waste stabilization ponds, wastewater storage and treatment reservoirs and constructed wetlands.

Maturation pond – An aerobic pond with algal growth and high levels of bacterial removal; usually the final type of pond in a waste stabilization pond system.

Median – The middle value of a sample series (50% of the values in the sample are lower and 50% are greater than the median).

Membrane filtration – Filtration technique based on a physical barrier (a membrane) with specific pore sizes that traps contaminants larger than the pore size on the top surface of the membrane. Contaminants smaller than the specified pore size may pass through the membrane or may be captured within the membrane by some other mechanism.

Metacercariae (infective) – Life cycle stage of trematode parasites infective to humans. Metacercariae can form cysts in fish muscle tissue or on the surfaces of plants, depending on the type of trematode species.

Multiple barriers – Use of more than one preventive measure as a barrier against hazards.

Nightsoil – Untreated excreta transported without water, e.g. via containers or buckets; often used as a popular term in an unspecific manner to designate faecal matter of any origin; its technical use is therefore not recommended.

Off-site sanitation – System of sanitation where excreta are removed from the plot occupied by the dwelling and its immediate surroundings.

On-site sanitation – System of sanitation where the means of storage are contained within the plot occupied by the dwelling and its immediate surroundings. For some systems (e.g. double-pit or vault latrines), treatment of the faecal matter happens on site also, through extended in-pit consolidation and storage. With other systems (e.g. septic tanks, single-pit or vault installations), the sludge has to be collected and treated off site (see also faecal sludge).

Oocyst – A structure that is produced by some coccidian protozoa (i.e. *Cryptosporidium*) as a result of sexual reproduction during the life cycle. The oocyst is usually the infectious and environmental stage, and it contains sporozoites. For the enteric protozoa, the oocyst is excreted in the faeces.

Operational monitoring – The act of conducting a planned sequence of observations or measurements of control parameters to assess whether a control measure is operating within design specifications (e.g. for wastewater treatment turbidity). Emphasis is given to monitoring parameters that can be measured quickly and easily and that can indicate if a process is functioning properly. Operational monitoring data should help managers to make corrections that can prevent hazard break-through.

Overhanging latrine – A latrine that empties directly into a pond or other water body.

Pathogen – A disease-causing organism (e.g. bacteria, helminths, protozoa and viruses).

pH – An expression of the intensity of the basic or acid condition of a liquid.

Policy – The set of procedures, rules and allocation mechanisms that provide the basis for programmes and services. Policies set priorities and often allocate resources for their implementation. Policies are implemented through four types of policy instruments: laws and regulations; economic measures; information and education programmes; and assignment of rights and responsibilities for providing services.

Primary treatment – Initial treatment process used to remove settleable organic and inorganic solids by sedimentation and floating substances (scum) by skimming. Examples of primary treatment include primary sedimentation, chemically enhanced primary sedimentation and upflow anaerobic sludge blanket reactors.

Quantitative microbial risk assessment (QMRA) – Method for assessing risk from specific hazards through different exposure pathways. QMRA has four components: hazard identification; exposure assessment; dose–response assessment; and risk characterization.

Regulations – Rules created by an administrative agency or body that interpret the statute(s) setting out the agency's purpose and powers or the circumstances of applying the statute.

Restricted irrigation – Use of wastewater to grow crops that are not eaten raw by humans.

Risk – The likelihood of a hazard causing harm in exposed populations in a specified time frame, including the magnitude of that harm.

Risk assessment – The overall process of using available information to predict how often hazards or specified events may occur (likelihood) and the magnitude of their consequences.

Risk management – The systematic evaluation of the wastewater, excreta or greywater use system, the identification of hazards and hazardous events, the assessment of risks and the development and implementation of preventive strategies to manage the risks.

Secondary treatment – Wastewater treatment step that follows primary treatment. Involves the removal of biodegradable dissolved and colloidal organic matter using high-rate, engineered aerobic biological treatment processes. Examples of secondary treatment include activated sludge, trickling filters, aerated lagoons and oxidation ditches.

Septage – Sludge removed from septic tanks.

Septic tank – An underground tank that treats wastewater by a combination of solids settling and anaerobic digestion. The effluents may be discharged into soak pits or small-bore sewers.

Sewage – Mixture of human excreta and water used to flush the excreta from the toilet and through the pipes; may also contain water used for domestic purposes.

Sewer – A pipe or conduit that carries wastewater or drainage water.

Sewerage – A complete system of piping, pumps, basins, tanks, unit processes and infrastructure for the collection, transporting, treating and discharging of wastewater.

Sludge – A mixture of solids and water that settles to the bottom of latrines, septic tanks and ponds or is produced as a by-product of wastewater treatment (sludge produced from the treatment of municipal or industrial wastewater is not discussed in this volume).

Source separation – Diversion of urine, faeces, greywater or all, followed by separate collection (and treatment).

Subsurface irrigation – Irrigation below the soil surface; prevents contamination of aboveground parts of crops

Surface water – All water naturally open to the atmosphere (e.g. rivers, streams, lakes and reservoirs).

Thermotolerant coliforms – Group of bacteria whose presence in the environment usually indicates faecal contamination; previously called faecal coliforms.

Tolerable daily intake (TDI) – Amount of toxic substance that can be taken on a daily basis over a lifetime without exceeding a certain level of risk

Tolerable health risk – Defined level of health risk from a specific exposure or disease that is tolerated by society, used to set health-based targets.

Turbidity – The cloudiness of water caused by the presence of fine suspended matter.

Ultraviolet radiation (UV) – Light waves shorter than visible blue-violet waves of the spectrum (from 380 to 10 nanometres) used for pathogen inactivation (bacteria, protozoa and viruses).

Unrestricted irrigation – The use of treated wastewater to grow crops that are normally eaten raw.

Upflow anaerobic sludge blanket reactor – High-rate anaerobic unit used for the primary treatment of domestic wastewater. Wastewater is treated during its passage through a sludge layer (the sludge "blanket") composed of anaerobic bacteria. The treatment process is designed primarily for the removal of organic matter (biochemical oxygen demand).

Validation – Testing the system and its individual components to prove that it is capable of meeting the specified targets (i.e. microbial reduction targets). Should take place when a new system is developed or new processes are added.

Vector – Insect that carries disease from one animal or human to another (e.g. mosquitoes).

Vector-borne disease – Diseases that can be transmitted from human to human via insects (e.g. malaria).

Verification monitoring – The application of methods, procedures, tests and other evaluations, in addition to those used in operational monitoring, to determine compliance with the system design parameters and/or whether the system meets specified requirements (e.g. microbial water quality testing for *E. coli* or helminth eggs, microbial or chemical analysis of irrigated crops).

Waste-fed aquaculture – Use of wastewater, excreta and/or greywater as inputs to aquacultural systems.

Waste stabilization ponds (WSP) – Shallow basins that use natural factors such as sunlight, temperature, sedimentation, biodegradation, etc., to treat wastewater or faecal sludges. Waste stabilization pond treatment systems usually consist of anaerobic, facultative and maturation ponds linked in series.

Wastewater – Liquid waste discharged from homes, commercial premises and similar sources to individual disposal systems or to municipal sewer pipes, and which contains mainly human excreta and used water. When produced mainly by household and commercial activities, it is called domestic or municipal wastewater or domestic sewage. In this context, domestic sewage does not contain industrial effluents at levels that could pose threats to the functioning of the sewerage system, treatment plant, public health or the environment.

Withholding period – Time to allow pathogen die-off between waste application and harvest.